Dance, Turn, Hop, Learn!

ALSO BY CONNIE BERGSTEIN DOW

One, Two, What Can I Do? Dance and Music for the Whole Day

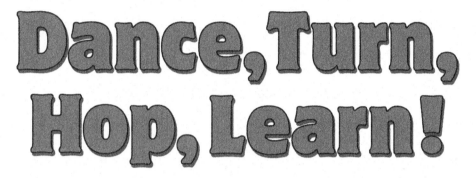

Dance, Turn, Hop, Learn!

Enriching Movement Activities for Preschoolers

Connie Bergstein Dow

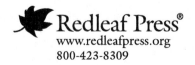
Redleaf Press®
www.redleafpress.org
800-423-8309

Published by Redleaf Press
10 Yorkton Court
St. Paul, MN 55117
www.redleafpress.org

First edition 2006
Cover illustration by Meredith Johnson
Interior typeset in H&FJ Whitney and designed by Percolator
Interior illustrations by Chris Wold Dyrud
Printed in the United States of America

Library of Congress Cataloging-in-Publication Data
Dow, Connie Bergstein.
    Dance, turn, hop, learn! : enriching movement activities for preschoolers / Connie Bergstein Dow.
        p. cm.
    Includes index.
    ISBN 978-1-929610-89-1
    1. Movement education. 2. Education, Preschool—Activity programs.   I. Title.
    GV452.D69 2006
    372.86—dc22
                                                                                                          2006012599

Printed on acid-free paper   U15-06

To my husband, Buzz, and my children,
David, Michael, and Jessica

Dance, Turn, Hop, Learn!

Acknowledgments

I have been fortunate to be surrounded by supportive family, friends, and colleagues during my career as a dancer and dance educator, as well as throughout the process of writing this book. I want to start at the beginning and thank my parents, Mary and Frank Bergstein, for the many opportunities they have given me throughout my life, and for introducing me to the world of art and dance.

Special teachers and mentors who guided me in my dance journey include Susan Alexander, Norah Parisi, Gay Delanghe, Vera Embree, Lisa Nowak, Jefferson James, Fanchon Shur, Daniel Simmons, and Nancy Fountain.

A particular thank-you goes to Kathleen L. Smith and L'Ana Burton of the Creative Dance Continuum, in New London, Connecticut, who graciously shared lesson ideas, specifically the dance code and the found objects bag. Jeanne Speier, dance therapist and dance teacher, lent her idea of the clothespin butterflies to use as playful props. The teaching skills, creativity, and love of dance shown by these professionals have been an inspiration to me.

Christopher Watson, artistic director of the Christopher Watson Dance Company, and director of Professional Development and Education at the Center for Early Education and Development at the University of Minnesota, encouraged my writing and first told me about Redleaf Press.

Catherine Burns, registered somatic movement therapist, and Jane Skinner Peck, dance educator (MAEd), reviewers extraordinaire, spent many hours going over the manuscript and communicating with me via long conference calls. I am forever grateful for their hard work, and the expertise and wonderful ideas they brought to the book.

Lynn Slaughter, dancer, teacher, writer, and long-time friend, encouraged me from the very beginning when the book was only an idea, and continued to be a mentor to me throughout the entire process. Ann Stewart, another special friend and writer, gave large doses of moral support, suggestions, and invaluable help. Other friends who have shown interest and unwavering faith in this project include Vicki Porter-Fink, Bruce Petrie Jr., Jane Friedman, and Judy Hollander. Mimi Brodsky Chenfeld, dance educator and author, has been a mentor in the short time I have had the pleasure of knowing her.

My sister, Martha Marcom, educator and co-founder of Yoga on High in Columbus, Ohio, has always shown unfaltering support of my dancing and my writing. My late brother, Tom Bergstein, was a wonderful musician and songwriter, and I continue to be inspired by his music and creative spirit.

All of the people with whom I have worked at Redleaf Press deserve an enormous thank-you. I am grateful for the faith they have had in this book from the beginning, and for all of the guidance they have offered throughout the writing process. Amanda Hane, development editor, who served as my editor, has been a constant source of encouragement, enthusiasm, and expertise. On top of that, Amanda never failed to answer my e-mailed questions almost instantaneously, and always cheerfully. I would also like to thank Sid Farrar, editor in chief, who brought me on board and provided constant support.

Much of the inspiration for this book has come from the many children I have had the pleasure of teaching over the years. I am in awe of their unending well of imagination and creative energy, and their capacity for expressing joy and wonder through movement.

My most important debt is to my family. My loving husband, Buzz, has been by my side for over thirty years. He has been as unwavering in his support of this book as he has been of my career as a dancer, teacher, and mother. My sons, David and Michael, and my daughter, Jessica, are a part of everything I do, and their energy, enthusiasm, and compassion are a part of this book as well. My love for my family is truly beyond words; it is to them I dedicate this book.

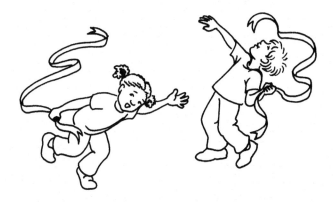

Introduction

During the thirty-five years that I have taught movement classes in public and private schools, teachers have often approached me and expressed interest in bringing creative movement into their own classrooms. But they have always quickly added that they didn't know where to start, or that they didn't know how to present movement concepts in an organized way. From the outset, the enthusiasm and interest of these teachers have been a primary inspiration for me. This book has been written for all those teachers of preschool children and child care providers who have wanted to bring movement into their classrooms but weren't sure where to begin.

For teachers with no formal dance training, the idea of bringing structured movement into a classroom may be daunting. Movement traditionally has not been as widely used in classrooms as other art forms, such as music, visual art, and drama, and many teachers may not know where to begin. In fact, movement is very accessible, and requires almost no materials. With a small drum or tambourine, a few recorded musical selections, a classroom space, and a guided lesson plan, you can present a playful, imaginative, and enriching class to your students.

I have found that the most difficult part of teaching a preschool movement class is not teaching the movement skills themselves, but learning how to work with young children. Because teachers are already familiar with handling a classroom full of young children, incorporating structured movement into the lesson plan can be a very straightforward process. In fact, it is a natural addition to the curriculum because young children love to move, and movement then becomes another helpful instructional tool for the teacher.

Dance, Turn, Hop, Learn! is designed to bridge the gap for teachers who recognize that movement can be a valuable tool in the classroom but who are not familiar with teaching structured movement classes. The thirty-eight lessons in this book will take you through a year of movement exploration and imagination and will give you the confidence to make creative movement a basic part of your classroom.

Movement Is Learning

Movement is one of the most basic and natural ways that children explore their surroundings. Every time a child moves, she is learning about her world. When a child drops a block and sees it fall to the floor, he is learning about gravity. When she plays with a doll, she is learning about social roles and about caring and nurturing. In the simple act of doing, the child is learning. All learning is first experiential and then conceptual. And much experiential learning for young children is done with their own bodies through their everyday physical interactions with their environment.

In the creative dance class, children explore different ways of moving and try on many different roles. In doing so, the child is learning how different parts of her body work, refining her large and fine motor skills, and beginning to understand concepts in the physical world such as speed, energy, and spatial orientation. The child is also practicing social skills such as listening, following directions, learning body control, and participating in a group activity. Movement can also serve as a springboard for learning about other subjects such as nature, communities, reading, and counting.

In addition, with the increasing emphasis placed on physical fitness as rates of childhood obesity rise, structured movement classes can be a wonderful way to teach children that movement and exercise can be fun and exciting. In many early child care environments, the large motor skills practice is limited to outside play or other open spaces for running and jumping. Bringing organized movement into the classroom can help children appreciate all the ways their bodies can move and make movement throughout the day a natural part of their lives.

So how can creative movement help a child in his journey of learning about the world? Because movement and learning are interwoven concepts in a young child's life, it follows that the use of structured movement in the classroom can be a positive, nurturing influence in a child's development. This exploration of the principles of movement, guided by the teacher, stimulates the children to engage in active, imaginative play, which leads to physical, intellectual, emotional, and creative growth.

PHYSICAL DEVELOPMENT

Within structured movement classes, the teacher can help to promote the development of young children's physical skills. This can be accomplished by channeling the child's love of movement into a specific activity. Creative movement classes are a time for children to do the things they already love to do, such as run, jump, turn, and move to music. A teacher might introduce a new skill by tapping into the child's love of one of these movements that he has already mastered. For example, a teacher can use the child's love of running, and guide the child to master a more complex and refined type of run, such as a gallop. The classes in this book help to lay a foundation for teaching and refining children's motor skills, while at the same time making the learning process enjoyable.

A very important component of children's physical development is learning how to control their own bodies. There is no better way for children to learn this self-control than in a structured movement class. This body control is not only important for children, it is a social skill that, when mastered by the students,

ultimately contributes to a more positive classroom environment for the students and teacher. When children are in a structured movement class, they learn the range of movement of the parts of their bodies, and they learn that they have a personal space of their own, within which they are moving. They learn that other children also have a personal space, and that those boundaries should be respected. They become accustomed to listening, processing the instructions, and, finally, incorporating the movement instructions into their own bodies. They learn to slow down and stop, control the speed at which they move, change directions in space, and respect the other children who are also moving at the same time in close proximity.

When children master these basic concepts in the creative movement class, the teacher then has a set of classroom management tools that can be incorporated into all aspects of the educational environment. The teacher will be guided in the book's first seven lesson plans as to how to introduce the classroom management techniques and basic movement skills, and these important body control concepts will be repeated and reinforced throughout the remaining lesson plans.

INTELLECTUAL DEVELOPMENT

The teacher can use movement as a means of fostering intellectual growth. Movement can be used to address almost any subject. Children can often understand abstract concepts more easily if they experience the concept in their own bodies. For example, the mathematical concept of subtraction can be demonstrated by placing children in a circle, counting aloud together how many children there are, and then having one child at a time sit down or come into the center of the circle. Early literacy concepts can also readily be addressed through movement. Poems, rhymes, books, and stories serve as lively accompaniments and stimuli for movement.

Creative movement classes can help children to make choices and search for solutions to problems through hands-on participation. The simple question "How can we change the way we walk?" can be solved in many different ways: change of direction, level, speed, rhythm, size of strides, or adding other body part movements to the walk (to name only some of the myriad possibilities). A child learns that there may not be just one way to answer a question or solve a problem, which then leads to the discovery of several solutions to a task or activity presented during the movement class. Through movement activities, children learn the concept that in many situations, there are no mistakes; there are only opportunities for many solutions. This attitude, when communicated to children, frees them to look for many answers as they approach a problem or task. They learn that often there isn't just one right and one wrong answer, but countless right answers.

Because movement is a concrete way for children to begin to grasp abstract or more complex ideas, movement classes are an excellent medium for addressing the early childhood learning standards. These goals may be broad concepts, such as mastering mathematic skills, or more specific ones, such as helping a child recognize and learn to move to rhythms. Each lesson in this book addresses one or more of the recognized national standards for early childhood learning. In this book, the Head Start Child Outcomes Framework is used as the guide for learning standards.

EMOTIONAL DEVELOPMENT

Throughout a creative dance lesson, the teacher presents ideas to the children for exploration. These tasks can have many different approaches and solutions. The children will experiment and solve them in individual ways, boosting their confidence, and thus their self-esteem. The children are given another means of expressing themselves; simply by moving, they can come up with creative solutions.

The teacher can further nurture the confidence-building benefits the children gain through solving the movement problems. A child who does not excel in verbal skills may shine in the arena of movement. If a teacher singles out this child, for example, when she comes up with a particularly imaginative answer to a movement task, she has a moment in the limelight and a boost of self-esteem, and her solution can serve as an inspiration to the other students. For example, a teacher might assign a task, such as "Can you find a way to move from one spot to another without touching the bottoms of your feet to the ground?" Then, if one of the children found a particularly creative solution, the teacher could bring the other students' attention to her and say something like "Look at Kia! She is crawling, and now she is scooting on her seat!

Kia, you came up with a great answer to my question!" In addition to helping to boost confidence, this kind of positive reinforcement also increases a child's interest in the subject. Singling a child out for praise in a movement class can be especially rewarding for one who is not progressing as quickly in other areas.

In addition, movement can give children another tool with which to express themselves. Children can learn that movement can be used to express emotions, focus their energy, and understand ideas. Children who have difficulty expressing themselves in words may thrive in a movement class. The ability to use many avenues to express feelings is a valuable tool in a child's emotional development.

CREATIVE DEVELOPMENT

Movement can be used as a springboard to stimulate a child's imagination. Simple questions, such as "What if you could fly? What would it feel like to be a bird? What do you think you could see if you were flying?" are easy and effective imagination-starters. The creative movement teacher can use movement prompts as teaching tools to encourage the children to move their bodies in a new way, as a lead-in to a game or story, or simply to allow the child to imagine himself in a new place or having a new experience. *Dance, Turn, Hop, Learn!* offers many suggestions for using movement to stimulate imagination, and draws on a variety of subjects that are interesting and enjoyable to preschoolers, using themes that loosely follow the school year.

It should also be noted that throughout the book the words *movement*, *creative movement*, and *dance* are interchangeable. Movement becomes art when it is used for something other than everyday tasks. Walking from one side of a room to the other is an everyday task. When a dancer walks dramatically from one side of the stage to the other, carefully controlling and directing his well-trained body, the movement has become art. The art form of dance uses the body and body movements as the medium of communication, just as music uses sound. In teaching a creative movement class, you are encouraging the children to think creatively about the ways in which they typically use their bodies. The components of dance provide a wealth of material for structuring classes and teaching children to use movement as a way to learn about their world.

How to Use This Book

This book consists of thirty-eight lessons that can be used each week throughout the school year. The lessons will take you through all the months of the year as you explore the different seasons and the themes that go along with them. However, it is not necessary to use the lessons in order. For example, you may want to pull out a lesson here or there that explores a theme you are studying with the class. These thirty-eight lessons can be used and adapted in any way that suits your setting, program, and/or curriculum.

The classes are designed for a maximum of ten children; larger groups can be accommodated as long as the child/teacher ratio is at least one teacher for every ten children. They are designed for children ages three to six. The children should dress for movement class in loose play clothes and soft-soled shoes or bare feet, but just as they play during recess in whatever they wore to school that day, they should be permitted to participate in the movement class even if they don't have the above-mentioned clothing.

CLASSROOM: NO TWO SPACES ARE ALIKE

The thirty-eight lessons can be adapted to any kind of classroom space. It is important to allow children some time during the school day for large, expansive movement. The classroom or child care setting may be limited in available space, but most of the activities in this book can be adapted to a small area. If there are objects in the middle of the room, such as bookshelves or tables, they can be incorporated right into the activity with the use of a little imagination and flexibility. For example, a table can be a central object to circle around while performing traveling movements; a bookshelf might be the boundary that signals a change of direction. Suggestions are given throughout the lessons in Part One for these types of spatial adaptations.

Of course, if a large, open space is available, with no objects or constraints, the lesson plans can be followed as written. The teacher and children will become accustomed to moving in whatever space is available to them and will find activities that work particularly well in their own classroom.

THE PROGRESSION OF THE LESSON PLANS: TEACHING THE TEACHER

The book is divided into two main parts. The first part introduces classroom management tools that will be helpful for leading movement classes. This part also presents the basic movement concepts that the children will be exploring throughout all the lessons in the book. Part Two then reinforces and expands the concepts introduced in Part One.

Part One, Lessons 1–7

Part One of the book includes the first seven lessons. Teaching the first seven lessons in order is the recommended approach to the book as the principal concepts for teaching movement are presented in a logical order; however, if the teacher is already comfortable using the lesson plans, the classes may be taught in the order that best suits his needs. Each of the seven lessons in Part One emphasizes specific classroom management tools and basic movement skills that will lay the groundwork for more smoothly functioning and structured movement classes in the future.

The classroom management tools are techniques that will enable the teacher to deal with the group of children, and help the children control their own bodies, so that learning can take place. The basic movement skills are principles of movement based on the tenets of the art of dance. These principles, such as body awareness, motor skills, and control of direction, speed, and energy, empower the children with the ability to control their bodies. The learning of these skills is one of the most important reasons that structured movement classes are beneficial in the early childhood classroom; the children learn body control, which is a win-win situation for both the students and the teacher. The classroom management tools and the basic movement skills are listed at the beginning of this part of the book.

Part Two, Lessons 8–38

Part Two encompasses the remaining thirty-one lesson plans. These are complete sessions built around the general theme of the lesson title. These thirty-one lessons are to be used once the first seven lessons have been completed, thus the classroom management tools and basic movement skills have all been systematically introduced, or if the teacher is already comfortable teaching movement. The more complex motor skills, such as gallops, are introduced in Part Two.

THE STRUCTURE OF THE LESSON PLANS

The principal objective of this book is to help the teacher introduce movement, as a teaching tool, to the classroom. The book is designed so that the teacher can easily access the material, know the goal of a specific activity, and then have directions and a script to guide the children through the activity to accomplish the goal.

Music and Materials:

Music and movement are natural companions and essential partners in a movement class for children. The lesson plan provides general musical style suggestions so that a teacher can draw from readily available resources. A few recommended CDs that will carry you through most of the activities in this book are highlighted in the index of music titles. Most of the lessons also have suggestions for specific selections that will complement and enhance the theme. All of the music titles are current and should be available at the local library. However, it is not necessary to have the exact selections listed in order for the class to be successful; it is more important that the children frequently have the opportunity to dance to musical accompaniment.

Many of the lessons also employ the use of simple materials for props such as scarves, clothespins, and stuffed animals. In addition, a number of the lessons are based on storybooks that can be found in your local library, or involve crafts that can easily be made with materials found in most early childhood classrooms. The materials needed for each lesson are listed and described for the teacher at the beginning of each lesson plan. As with the musical selections, though, it is not always necessary to have the exact materials. If you do not have the recommended books or stories, you may bring in pictures instead that highlight the theme of the day. Variations are suggested throughout the lessons. In addition, if you do not have the exact materials that the lesson requires, you can come up with your own adaptations using a little creativity and imagination!

Early Childhood Learning Standards:

The lessons in this book are all correlated with one or more of the Head Start early childhood learning stan-

dards. As noted above, movement classes in the early childhood classroom not only are a great way to develop the children's large motor skills, but can provide the foundation for learning in a number of different domains. In each lesson, you will find listed the early childhood learning standards that will be addressed in the activities in the lesson. These are then indexed at the back of the book.

The Lesson Description:

The Lesson Description is the actual text that guides the teacher through the different parts of the class. In order for a teacher to feel comfortable following the lesson plans in this book, it is important to understand the flow and structure of a movement/dance class. A movement class usually consists of four major components, which are the warm-up, the large motor skills practice, the body of the class, and the conclusion. The classes in this book are based on this structure, but the sections have been tailored to the preschool-aged child, and are described below.

Each of the four sections is clearly delineated and includes the preparation and script for presentation of the activities. Throughout the lesson plan, italics are used when there are suggested words, explanations, or stories that the teacher can use while presenting the lesson.

1. Opening Activity

The introductory activity in each lesson is an opportunity to immediately focus the children's attention on movement. It also serves the purpose of allowing them to be active right away, instead of having to sit quietly and await the beginning of class. Usually children come into the open space of a classroom and begin moving right away anyway, so a loosely structured improvisation is a way of warming up their bodies and easing them into the more structured sections of the class.

2. Greeting Circle

The purpose of the Greeting Circle is to provide a transition between the Opening Activity and the Movement Exploration. The teacher can use this time to greet the children and briefly discuss the lesson theme.

3. Movement Exploration

In this section of the lesson, movement games, improvisations, stories, and prop explorations are introduced that are based on the theme for the day. This is an opportunity for the teacher to cultivate the children's imaginations, while at the same time address the lesson goals. Musical accompaniment is often a very important enhancement to the activities of this section of the class.

The teacher can also use this part of the class to introduce and practice seated warm-up exercises and large motor skills with the children. The majority of the classes in this book begin the Movement Exploration with a seated warm-up. These are short exercises, designed specifically for young children, to guide them in warming up different parts of their bodies. The seated warm-ups are then followed by the large motor skills practice. For this part of the class, the children line up on one side of the classroom and practice different large motor skills such as walking, running, and galloping as they travel together to the other side of the room. The motor skills are introduced individually in the earlier lessons and reinforced throughout the remaining lessons. Both the seated warm-ups and the motor skills practices are presented in a playful way, using the lesson theme, so that the repetition of the skills is both fun and challenging for the children.

4. Good-Bye Circle

There is almost always a quiet finish to a dance class, no matter how strenuous and exciting it has been up to this point. In a creative movement lesson for young children, it is especially important to bring the children back to a calm state of mind after the stimulation of movement. Suggestions are given for ending each class, which will help to reinforce an idea or concept from the lesson theme.

The lessons are laid out in sections, and each one, if taught as a whole, will take about thirty minutes. Most of the sections in the four-part lesson plan will last about five to seven minutes each. Thus, you may want to choose only one section, or several sections of a lesson, and plug them into your own class plan for the day. After reading a book about a particular subject, pull out one or two sections from a lesson in this book with a related theme to the one you are teaching, and reinforce the learning of that theme with a movement activity. Or use part of one class and part of another, if that works better for your particular classroom goals. Used in this way, the book can increase the instructional tools you have at your disposal throughout the entire school year.

This book is a manual; it will be a work in progress to guide you through your journey of teaching movement. There is a space at the end of every lesson for you to write down what worked and what didn't work in each lesson. The students will probably generate as many ideas about the lesson theme as the book itself offers; take the opportunity to write the ideas down immediately, so they will be available to you the next time you teach that lesson or explore a related theme.

Once you have become comfortable with the flow of teaching a movement class, and see how adaptable the classes are to the learning environment, you may want to develop your own lesson plans. There may be ideas and themes you would like to present that are not covered in these thirty-eight lessons. A blank Lesson Plan Template is printed at the back of the book to be copied and used for new lesson ideas.

A NOTE ON CHILDREN WITH SPECIAL NEEDS

Children with special needs can actively participate in any of the movement activities with some simple adaptations. All children should have the opportunity to participate in whatever capacity they can.

For children with physical disabilities, the teacher may need to increase the amount of space needed for the activities and remove barriers such as bookshelves and tables. The use of props, particularly if they are heavy, may need to be modified for the child to use them. The teacher should be particularly watchful for signs of fatigue or other signs of exertion. If a child is physically unable to perform an exercise, she may also be given a toy or doll with moveable body parts to manipulate according to the instructions.

For children with visual impairments, you may need to delineate the boundaries of the movement area with bright colors, and remove other impediments such as bookshelves or tables. Clear verbal instructions are particularly important for children with visual impairments, and you can also use sound in the form of drumbeats or musical changes to help the child recognize transitions. Having the child partner with another child can also be useful for a child with visual impairments.

Just as children with visual impairments respond to auditory cues, children with hearing impairments will respond well to visual cues. Demonstrating a movement first for the child can be particularly useful, as can having the child partner with another child during the exercise. The use of cue cards, props, and other signals such as turning the lights on and off to signal a transition may also be helpful.

Children with learning and emotional disabilities often do particularly well in movement classes because movement provides another tool for learning and self-expression. Clear, consistent instructions are important for a child with learning or emotional disabilities in this environment, as well as having minimal outside distractions. In addition, you may want to "shine the spotlight" on these children for solving problems creatively and provide plenty of positive reinforcement.

Children with special needs not only can participate, but they often thrive in a movement class. These lessons can easily be tailored and adapted to your own classroom environment to include all children in the movement activities.

Have Fun with This Book!

The driving force behind this book is my belief that creative dance, as well as the other arts, should be a part of every young child's life. Movement classes should be seen not only as a way to promote large motor skill development but also as the basis for all types of learning, from artistic expression to creative problem solving to social development. Once familiar with the use of this book, you can look forward to an exciting year, as you and your young students discover and explore the sheer joy of moving. The wonder that comes with exploring how their bodies move and the world around them is as valuable as anything else the children will learn in this book.

Have fun!

Part One

Lessons 1 through 7

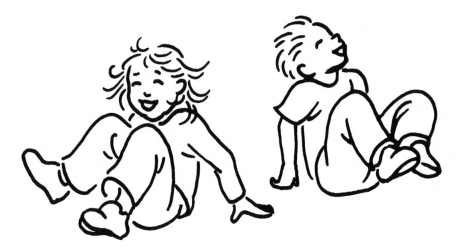

Introduction of Classroom Management Tools
and Basic Movement Skills

CLASSROOM MANAGEMENT TOOLS

Goal: Students will be introduced to the following important concepts for overall classroom protocol during the listed classes in Part One.

Listening to and Following Movement Instructions	(Lessons 1–7)
Cues for Stopping	(Lessons 1, 2, 3)
Personal Space and Shared Space	(Lessons 1, 2, 3)
Guidelines for Free Group Movement	(Lessons 2, 3, 4)
Group Cooperation and Taking Turns	(Lessons 3, 4, 5)
Guidelines for Working with Props	(Lessons 2, 6)
Shine the Spotlight	(Lessons 6, 7)

BASIC MOVEMENT SKILLS

Goal: Students will develop proficiency in age-appropriate movement skills and will learn to use creative movement as an approach to solving problems during the listed classes in Part One.

Control of Speed, or Tempo	(Lessons 1–7)
Control of Direction in Space (includes level, direction, floor pattern, size)	(Lessons 1, 2, 3, 4, 7)
Control of Energy (use of energy and flow to create a specific movement quality)	(Lessons 6, 7)
Body Awareness (includes body parts, balance, and shape)	(Lessons 1–7)
Problem Solving through Movement	(Lessons 1–7)
Locomotor Movements (moving from one place to another)	(Lessons 1–7)
Moving to Rhythms, Music, or Sounds	(Lessons 1–7)
Working with Props	(Lessons 2, 6)
Dramatic Play	(Lesson 5)
Sequencing (learning a series of movements)	(Lesson 5)

Moving by Myself and Moving with Friends

The lessons in this book are designed to create a safe and ordered, yet pleasant and fun, classroom environment. One of the most important gifts that movement classes can offer children and teachers is the tools with which to develop body control. This lesson is an introduction to the movement class for both the teacher and student.

These activities will also help familiarize the children with the concept of "personal space" versus "shared space." They will learn that personal space can be thought of not only as a specific spot on the floor to which they are assigned, but as a "bubble" of personal space that will travel with them throughout the classroom. This concept is very important, especially when the subsequent lessons begin to introduce more free group movement activities.

Shared space is the space in which all of the rest of the children are traveling throughout the room. This lesson will also help the children recognize and respect the "bubble" of space around the other children. These skills lay an important foundation for the child's social and emotional development.

MUSIC SUGGESTIONS:

General
- One upbeat instrumental musical selection or song

Specific Selection
- "Get Ready, Get Set, Let's Dance" (*Kids in Action*, Greg & Steve, Greg & Steve Productions, 2000)

MATERIALS NEEDED:
- Masking tape, or a small non-skid mat, one per child
- A large, portable drum (not required, but useful—a tambourine or small drum can be used in place of a large drum in all the lessons)

Early Learning Standards
1B, 17B, 18B, 19C, 24A, 25A*

* These standards will be integrated into every lesson as strategies for classroom management and for fostering movement skill. They will be explored in some way in every class, but as other goals will also be targeted, they will not be listed specifically in each lesson.

Opening Activity: Personal Space

1. Prepare the Space: Evenly throughout the available classroom space, assign a spot for each child. An "X" of masking tape or a small non-skid rug work well as a visual cue. This will help the children to become familiar with the idea of their own spots, and their accompanying personal spaces.

2. Assign the Spots: When the children come into the classroom, explain that each one will have his very own spot. You can assign designated spots, or allow the children to find their own. Tell the children that the spot on the floor is each one's own personal space.

3. Introduce the "Stop" Signal: Once the children are seated on their spots, you can introduce the "stop" signal. One loud, sharp drum or tambourine beat will mean that they should stop what they are doing, and turn their attention to the teacher. The signal can mean a change, transition, or end of an activity. The "stop" signal is specifically written into this lesson, but will not be written each time in future lessons.

4. Begin the Activity: Have the children stand on their spots. *Can you try moving up and down on your spot? Move as slowly as you can. Good! Now, every time I sound the loud drum beat, freeze right where you are!* Repeat until you have practiced the stop cue with the children several times.

5. Increase the Speed: *Can you move up and down more quickly? The drum beat still means that you have to stop right where you are!* Continue this activity, asking the children to increase the tempo of their up and down movement, until they have learned to stop on cue. Allow the children to increase their speed only to the point that they can maintain body control while moving.

Teaching Tip: Remind the children to control their bodies when they quickly fall to the floor, catching themselves with their hands.

Greeting Circle

1. Walk in a Circle: *Now we will leave our spots and come together into a circle. Whenever we are standing or sitting closely in a circle, we want to try not to bump anyone near us. Let's walk around the circle, and see if we can keep the spaces between each other. When you hear the stop signal, freeze.*

2. Walk the Other Way: *Turn around and walk in the other direction now, still keeping the spaces between each other.* (stop signal at end)

3. Up and Down: *Your personal space is now right in the spot where you stopped walking. Let's try going up and down again on our spots in this circle.* Remind them to stay in their own space, not touching anyone. *Can you think of three different ways to go up and down?* Use the stop signal at the end.

Movement Exploration: On or Off the Spot

ON THE SPOT

Ask the children to sit on their spots from the opening activity, look around the room, and see where their spots are in relation to others.

1. Sitting and Turning: *Can you sit and turn without leaving your spot?* (stop signal) *Can you turn around the other way?* (stop signal)

2. Moving Arms and Legs: *Can you move your arms and legs while sitting on your spot?* (stop signal)

3. Standing and Sitting: *Can you stand up and sit down?* (stop signal)

4. Standing and Turning: *Can you stand up and then turn around? The other way?* (stop signal)

5. Jumping and Hopping: *Can you jump up and down on your spot?* (stop signal) *Can you hop?* (stop signal)

6. Balancing: *Can you balance on one foot on your spot?* (stop signal)

You can do so many different movements while staying in one spot!

Teaching Tip: The activity "On or Off the Spot" requires only a small amount of space.

OFF THE SPOT

1. Back and Forth: *Let's take one step forward off the spot in any direction. Now take a backward step, and see that you are back on your spot!* (stop signal) Repeat this activity several times in many directions.

2. Jumping over the Spot: *Can you jump over your spot?* (stop signal) *Try jumping in different ways over your spot!* (stop signal)

3. Circling the Spot: *Can you circle around your spot? Now the other way?* (stop signal)

4. Circle Backward: *Circle your spot by taking backward steps. Look over your shoulder so you see where you are going as you move backward around your spot.* (stop signal)

5. Bigger Circles: *Let's try to make a bigger circle around our spots. Walk slowly in a circle around your spot, and let it become a little bigger each time. When you come very close to another person making her circle, stop and freeze!* They will freeze at different times. Remind them to hold the frozen position until everyone has frozen.

6. Point out Their Bubbles of Personal Space: *Look, everyone has stopped! Look back to see how far away you are from your own spot. Where you stopped is where* your personal space ends, and someone else's begins. Your own personal space is like a big bubble, and you are inside of it. See how big your bubble of personal space is?

7. Connecting the Bubbles of Personal Space: *Wave to the person nearest you, and then gently touch the person with your hand. Go back to your own spot. Go forward again, and gently touch the person's foot with your foot when your personal spaces touch. Try it again, touching elbows, and then touching backs. (stop signal)*

8. Bubble of Personal Space—Not Touching: *Now we will try something different. Go forward one more time, and come very close to the other person's bubble, but don't get close enough to touch the person. Imagine the bubble of space around him or her, and don't come into anyone else's bubble. Now go back to your spot.* Repeat this several times, in different directions.

9. Sum It Up: Sum up the importance of what was explored during this activity: *This is good practice for how we learn to move together. We can come close to others, but we don't want to touch their bubbles. When I talk about someone's bubble or personal space, that means you will try not to move so close to someone that you bump into him. Always respect the personal space of the others when we are moving together in our shared space.*

DO YOU REMEMBER WHERE YOUR SPOT IS?

For a game that will determine if they have learned where their own spots are, ask all the students to go to a specific place in the room, such as a corner. Assign them a type of movement to do that will take them back to their spots:

Take giant steps to your spot, being careful not to touch anyone else. Remember your bubble and everyone else's while you are walking. When you get to your own spot, jump three times. (Use the stop signal once they all jump three times.)

Variation: Replace giant steps with baby steps, side steps, tiptoe steps.

DANCE ON YOUR SPOT

Play the song "Get Ready, Get Set, Let's Dance," or other upbeat music, and allow the children to do a free dance on their spots within their bubbles of space. Prompt them to play with the ideas from this class: up and down on the spot, back and forth in different directions in the bubble, circle the spot, and jump over the spot.

Good-Bye Circle

Let's stand in a circle and see if we can go down to the floor within our own bubbles one more time. Now let's wave good-bye to each other while we are sitting in our bubbles! Can you wave with other parts of your body, like your elbow, your knee, your shoulder, your head, your foot?

Notes

What was successful about this lesson?

Which ideas could have worked better? How could they be improved?

What ideas were generated by the children during the lesson?

How would you enhance or expand this lesson in the future?

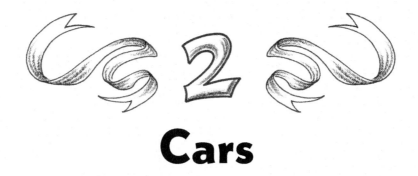

Cars

In this activity, the children will imagine they are driving cars, and can practice control of speed and direction while moving freely together. In addition, this activity is designed to reinforce the concepts of personal space and shared space that were addressed in Lesson 1. This activity is also a great opportunity to encourage the children's language development. The children will be building their vocabularies as they translate words like *up*, *down*, *inside*, and *outside* into action.

MUSIC SUGGESTIONS:

General

- Upbeat instrumental music, one slow, one faster
- Any music that starts slowly and changes to a fast tempo

Specific Selection

- "Beep Beep" (*Playmates Golden Classics*, Collectibles, 1991)

MATERIALS NEEDED:

- Drum or other portable percussion instrument
- Optional: Masking tape, or a small non-skid mat, one per child
- Optional: Plastic keys from baby toy key rings, one per child

Early Learning Standards
9E, 18B

Opening Activity: Where Can I Go in My Bubble?

Ask the children to start on their spots, either the ones from Lesson 1 or new ones you have designated. Use masking tape or non-skid mats again if the children need the visual cue to remember their spots. Remind the children that they will each be inside their own bubble of personal space during this activity.

1. Around: Ask the children to walk a circle around their spots, without touching anyone. Then ask them to walk that same circle backward, looking over their shoulders. The circle that they have just walked, without touching anyone else, is the size of their bubble for this activity.

2. Many directions from the center: Ask the children: *Can you go inside to the center of your bubble? Can you go out to the edge of your bubble? Now go back to the center, and choose another direction and go to the edge. Remember, the edge of your bubble is as far as you can go without touching another person.* Repeat this so that they have explored the edges of the bubble in all directions.

3. Up: *Can you reach up to the top of your bubble? Feel the round shape of it by standing on your tiptoes and reaching with your hands.*

4. Down: *Now, let's see how low our bubble is. Let's get down on the floor and find the bottom of the round shape.*

5. Inside and Outside: *Starting on your spot, do you think you could jump all the way to the edge of your bubble? It's a big jump! Jump out, and then turn around and jump back in! Let's try it in all directions from our spot.*

6. Across: Ask the children: *Can you jump all the way from one side of your bubble to the other?*

Variation: Try the above two with hopping.

Greeting Circle

This short activity will reinforce the body control concept of direction. Gather the children and have them stand in a circle. Explain that you are going to call each one's name, and as you do, you are going to assign them one of these direction ideas:

1. Around: *Walk around the circle, back to your original place in the circle.*

2. Up: *Stand up and reach as high as you can!*

3. Down: *Show us how low you can get to the floor.*

4. Inside: *Go inside to the center of the circle, and back to your place.*

5. Outside: *Walk a short distance away from the circle, and come back.*

6. Across: *Walk across and find a place on the other side of the circle.*

> **Teaching Tip:** *Pace your teaching based on the children's attention to and enjoyment of the activity.*

Movement Exploration: Cars

"Cars" is the first activity in which the children will be moving freely in the shared space. It is especially important for them to remember their bubbles, which are now their cars. Remind the children that they will try not to bump into anyone else's car, and they will try to control the speed and direction of their own cars. Running out of control is not part of this activity. They will need to drive safely!

1. Imagine Your Car: To begin the activity, instruct the children to return to their original spots, and pass out the plastic keys if you have brought them. Prompt them to imagine that their bubble is going to become a car, and they are each inside of their own car. *What color car would you imagine you are driving?*

> **Teaching Tip:** *Introduce the guidelines for using props. The children should not touch one another with the prop. They should use the prop only as instructed. They should hold onto it while moving and should not throw it or use it in any way that could damage it.*

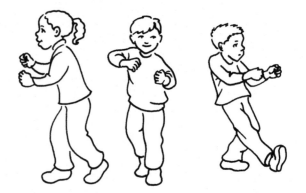

2. Drive Slowly: Play one of the slow musical selections. Explain that they will start walking slowly when the music begins: *Let's start our cars! Fasten your seat belt. Turn the key. Let's all be very careful drivers, and watch out for the other cars!*

3. Put on Your Brakes! Once the children are familiar with moving slowly in the space, have them practice stopping. A loud beat on the drum means that they should put on their brakes and wait for more instructions.

4. Direction Change: Next, introduce the idea of direction change after the stop. The loud beat will signal a stop, and once they have stopped for a few seconds, tell them that they will start up again, but going in a different direction. Repeat this stop and start game several times.

5. Speed Up: If this activity has worked well and there is more time, try it using a faster selection of music, and allowing the children to move at a faster pace (a fast walk or slow run; remind them that they must stay in control of their speed). Another option is to play "Beep Beep," or a selection that begins slowly and gradually increases in tempo.

6. Slow Down and Park Your Car: At the end of the activity, ask the children to put on their brakes to slow down, and park their cars in their original spots. *Take off your seat belt and turn your key to turn off the engine!*

Good-Bye Circle

Let's make a circle, with space in between each other. Now, let's walk slowly toward the center, closing the space between each other until we are touching hands with our arms open wide. Hold your neighbors' hands, and let's bow all together toward the center of the circle.

Notes

What was successful about this lesson?

Which ideas could have worked better? How could they be improved?

What ideas were generated by the children during the lesson?

How would you enhance or expand this lesson in the future?

Stoplights and Winding Roads

This lesson consists of two main activities. The first, a stoplight game, continues the theme of personal space from Lesson 2 as the children further practice controlling their direction and speed. The second activity is a simple obstacle course, which will challenge the children in following step-by-step instructions. In addition, this activity is designed for one or two children at a time, so the children will be introduced to the concept of waiting their turns to go through the course. Finally, as in the last lesson, the children will continue to build on their vocabulary of directional words.

MUSIC SUGGESTIONS:

General
- Upbeat instrumental music or songs

Specific Selections
- "Dance in Your Pants" (*Dance in Your Pants*, David Jack, Ta-Dum Productions, 2002)
- "The Entertainer" (*The Complete Rags of Scott Joplin*, Music Masters Jazz, 1995)

MATERIALS NEEDED:

- Three large (about 9 inches in diameter) cardboard or construction paper cut-outs of circles—one red, one yellow, one green, and an optional blue circle
- Items in the classroom that could be used for an obstacle course, such as tables, chairs, bookshelves, rug squares, or plastic cones
- Drum or other portable percussion instrument

Early Learning Standards
9E, 19C

Begin this activity by asking the children to find a personal space (it can be the one from the first two lessons, or you can ask them to choose new ones).

1. Introduce the Activity: Ask the children if they are familiar with stoplight colors. Show them the green cardboard circle, which will signal "go," yellow for "slow down," and red for "stop." Explain that you are the stoplight , and they will need to watch you carefully. "Dance in Your Pants" or a long song of upbeat music is a good accompaniment for this activity.

2. Direct the Traffic: Once the children are in their chosen spots, prompt them to imagine that their bubble of space is a car, just as they did in the last lesson. Standing in an area near the center of the space, hold up the green circle and prompt the children to begin moving in their imaginary cars. After a short time, randomly switch the colors one by one, making sure the children have followed the movement or stop signal before switching to another signal. Finish with the red light to signal the end of the activity.

 Teaching Tip: Remind the children to move in control, imagining their car as their bubble of space.

Variation: Once the children have mastered the above game, repeat it with the addition of the blue cardboard circle. This can signal "change of direction."

Greeting Circle

Bring the children together in a circle and ask, *What are some other signals that mean "stop"? Have you ever seen the flashing lights at a train crossing? A stop sign? A police officer directing traffic? And remember that my loud drum beat is also a stop signal!*

Movement Exploration: Obstacle Course

For this activity, you will be setting up an obstacle course using items you already have in the classroom, such as tables, chairs, bookshelves, plastic blocks, cones, and rug squares. Make the "road" have a set path that winds around and try to incorporate all different directional cues such as *under* a table, *over* a bridge, or *inside* a circle of masking tape.

> **Teaching Tip:** *If you have a large number of children, set up more than one obstacle course and use them simultaneously.*

1. Demonstrate the Course: Before the children go through the course, explain the sequence of the obstacles, using direction words (up, down, around, inside, outside, across, and through) as you demonstrate the course.

2. Take Turns: Assemble the children at the beginning of the "road." An upbeat musical accompaniment would work well during this activity, such as "The Entertainer," but play it quietly so you can direct with your voice. Several children can go through the course at once, but start them in intervals, leaving enough time between each one so that they will not get too close to each other. Again, remind them that they must control their speed and direction in order to get through the course. Use the stop cue at any time during this activity.

Variation: Instruct them to try going through the obstacle course in the reverse direction, starting at the end and going back to the beginning.

Good-Bye Circle

Stand in the middle of the good-bye circle with the colored circles. Ask the children to bow according to your signal:

Green:	Bow quickly toward the center
Yellow:	Bow slowly toward the center
Blue:	Bow away from the circle
Red:	Freeze

Randomly change the signals, and finish with the red stop signal.

Notes

What was successful about this lesson?

Which ideas could have worked better? How could they be improved?

What ideas were generated by the children during the lesson?

How would you enhance or expand this lesson in the future?

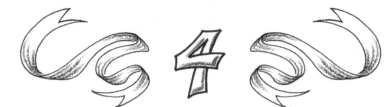

Trains, Boats, and Airplanes

This is a lesson about the many ways we go from one place to another. The first activity addresses how we move ourselves, and the following ones address different machines that take us from place to place. This lesson is designed to help children further develop their ability to discern similarities and differences among objects, in this case, forms of transportation. In addition, the children will continue to practice moving together freely in a shared space.

MUSIC SUGGESTIONS:

General
- Music about forms of transportation
- Upbeat instrumental music

Specific Selections
- "On My Way to School" (*Mother Earth*, Tom Chapin, Gadfly, 2001)
- "Riding in an Airplane" (*One Light One Sun*, Raffi, Rounder/Pgd, 1996)
- "Under the Sea" (*Little Mermaid Original Motion Picture Soundtrack*, Disney, 1997)
- "I've Been Working on the Railroad" (*Children's Favorites*, Various Artists, Music for Little People, 1997)
- "Peace Train" (*When Bullfrogs Croak*, Zak Morgan, Zak Records, 2003)

MATERIALS NEEDED:
- Drum or other portable percussion instrument
- Pictures of trains, boats, and airplanes

Early Learning Standards
11B

Opening Activity: Moving Ourselves

This activity is another opportunity to practice free group movement. Remind the children of the guidelines for free movement: they should control their bodies and move within their own bubble of personal space, while still respecting the personal space of others.

Free Movement Improvisation: Start with a free movement improvisation to a musical selection that highlights different ways of moving, such as Tom Chapin's "On My Way to School." If you don't have this particular musical selection, simply call out different ways of moving while music is playing, such as walk, march, tiptoe, hop, jump, turn, and crawl, demonstrating if necessary.

Greeting Circle

We moved ourselves in the last activity using different parts of our bodies. Can you think of some other ways that people go from place to place? In the last lesson we danced about cars. Are there other machines that carry people? Machines that help us move from place to place are called "transportation."

Movement Exploration: Transportation

SEATED WARM-UP

Have the children sit in a circle and introduce these exercises to illustrate the many different machines that transport us. Seated exercises will be used in many lessons throughout the book. Each exercise can be repeated several times as long as the children are interested.

1. Merry-Go-Round: Seated with knees close to the chest, use the arms to twirl around two or three times. Repeat, turning to the other side. Remind the children that the merry-go-round is a form of transportation.

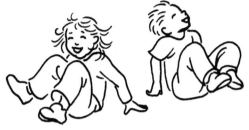

2. Boat: Seated with soles of feet together and knees apart, rock side to side and ask, *Where would you like to imagine you are going in your boats?* Start by rocking gently, then gradually increase the size and energy of the swaying.

3. Bring the Children to Standing: Suggest to the children that they lie face down on the floor, and imagine first that they are a submarine, and then that they are going to shoot into space like a rocket.

4. Pogo-Stick: Ask the children to jump around the room, imagining they are on a pogo stick—another form of transportation!

5. Conclude the Activity: *We have already danced about a merry-go-round, a boat, a submarine, a rocket, and a pogo stick! There are so many kinds of transportation, and we will dance about more!*

TRAINS, BOATS, AND AIRPLANES

The next three activities are an exploration of three kinds of transportation. They all use space, speed, and direction in different ways.

1. Trains: Gather the children together in a circle and discuss this form of transportation: *Does a train travel on the land? Do you know that its wheels go on tracks? Does it carry lots of people? Can it travel slowly? Fast? Have you ever seen one?* If you have any pictures of trains, you can show these to the children.

Now help the students make their own "train." Divide them up into groups of three or four, and have each trio or quartet make a train by standing in a line. Give each child a task: ring the bell, drive the train, honk the horn, look out the window.

Play the music, and prompt them to start moving slowly, staying in a line and following their leader. "I've Been Working on the Railroad" or "Peace Train" are good accompaniments to this activity. Later, signal them to stop, and ask them to change places within their line until each has had a turn at all of the tasks.

2. Boats: Gather the children together again and talk about boats and how they differ from cars and trains. Show the children any pictures you have brought of different kinds of boats.

For the boat activity, delineate a small area in the center of the room, which is the "boat." The song "Under the Sea" works well with this movement improvisation. Have the children sit in the "boat" and begin by swaying together gently. Imagine that the waves get bigger, sway even more, and encourage the children to roll off the boat and pretend to swim. As the children are swimming in the ocean, prompt them to share what they see. Finish this game with everyone back on the boat.

3. Airplanes: Gather the children back together in a circle and discuss how airplanes are different from boats and trains. If you have brought any pictures of airplanes, show these to the children.

Now have the children line up against one side of the space, and ask them to imagine they are the pilots of their own airplanes. Remind them that airplanes take off slowly, and then gain speed to get into the air. Once they are flying, play "Riding in an Airplane," or another selection of music, and encourage them to fly all around the room. Ask the children: *What does it feel like to be flying an airplane? What do you see? Where are you going?*

When it is time for them to land the planes, remind them that they will begin slowing down, and then will put on their brakes to come to a full stop.

 Teaching Tip: *Each child's bubble of personal space is now her imaginary airplane!*

Variation: If there is extra time, prompt the children to move freely as if they are using different forms of transportation such as a tractors, helicopters, dog sleds, roller skates, bicycles, or a school bus. Invite the children to move to their own ideas, or select one idea at a time and have the class improvise together.

Good-Bye Circle

Ask the children which form of transportation from today's class was their favorite. Suggest that each one use his or her favorite form of transportation to come together into the circle to say good-bye.

Notes

What was successful about this lesson?

Which ideas could have worked better? How could they be improved?

What ideas were generated by the children during the lesson?

How would you enhance or expand this lesson in the future?

Nursery Rhymes

Children enjoy moving to rhythm, and they especially like the familiar rhythms in classic nursery rhymes. Rhymes are a great way to help children learn to differentiate sounds and words, and in this lesson, the children will explore many rhymes and songs through movement. As they perform the nursery rhymes for the class, the children will also be practicing taking turns and cooperating as a group.

MUSIC SUGGESTIONS:

General
- Any recorded nursery rhymes or songs

Specific Selection
- "Head, Shoulders, Knees, and Toes" and "Jump Rope Medley" (*101 Toddler Favorites*, Various Artists, Music for Little People, 2003)

MATERIALS NEEDED:
- Clothespins or other small items for each child to jump over
- Drum

Early Learning Standards
4A, 3A, 3B, 3C, 13A

Opening Activity: Rhyming Games

1. Head, Shoulders, Knees, and Toes: Have the children stand with you in a circle. Either sing or play the recording of the song "Head, Shoulders, Knees, and Toes," and have the children touch the body parts as they are named in the song:

> *Head, shoulders, knees and toes, knees and toes*
> *Head, shoulders, knees and toes, knees and toes*
> *Eyes and ears and mouth and nose*
> *Head, shoulders, knees and toes, knees and toes.*

Practice this song until the children have mastered all the movements.

2. Rhyming Game: Now play a rhyming game about the body. Try this one, or make up your own. As in the last exercise, have the children touch each body part as it is named:

> *Head, toes, head, toes, let's all touch our nose!*
> *Head, back, head, back, do a jumping jack!*
> *Head, thigh, head, thigh, let's all pretend to cry!*
> *Head, hair, head, hair, let's point over there!*
> *Head, hip, head, hip, now, let's touch our lip!*
> *Head, face, head, face, let's all jump in place!*
> *Head, shoulders, go down low, now touch your elbow!*

The children can make up more rhymes, and you can encourage them to use as many body parts as possible.

3. Jump Rope Medley: Finish this warm-up section with the children pretending to jump rope to the songs in "Jump Rope Medley." If you don't have the recording, recite the jump rope rhyme "Miss Mary Mack" while the children jump:

> *Miss Mary Mack, Mack, Mack*
> *All dressed in black, black, black*
> *With silver buttons, buttons, buttons*
> *All down her back, back, back.*
>
> *She asked her mother, mother, mother*
> *For 50 cents, cents, cents*
> *To see the elephants, elephants, elephants*
> *Jump over the fence, fence, fence.*
>
> *They jumped so high, high, high*
> *They reached the sky, sky, sky*
> *And they didn't come back, back, back*
> *'Til the 4th of July, ly, ly!*

Greeting Circle

Bring the children together in a circle and ask them if they like to rhyme. Go around the circle, and help each child to think of a word that rhymes with his name, or the name of a pet, family member, or friend.

Movement Exploration: Nursery Rhymes

The remainder of the lesson will include many common nursery rhymes. Choose one to try first, and if there is time, choose another one!

1. Jack and Jill: Ask the children to recite "Jack and Jill" with you. Tell them: *Now we will dance it! Find a place on the floor.* Recite the rhyme slowly again as the children improvise movement through the different sections of the rhyme. *Imagine your hill. How can you climb up the hill? It is very steep. You have made it to the top! What can you see from up here? How would you fall down? How would you roll down the hill? Let's do it all together.*

2. Jack Be Nimble: Recite this rhyme once with the children. *Now, I will give each of you a "candlestick."* Hand out a clothespin or other small item to each child. *Try to jump over your "candlestick." Now try bouncing or clapping to the beat of the rhyme as we recite it. Make sure to jump over your candlestick when we get to that part!*

Variation: Change the word "jump" in this rhyme to "hop" or "jump backward."

3. Little Miss Muffet: Recite this rhyme all together. To dance this story, have two people at a time "perform," while the rest of the class is the audience. Each person in the pair should have a chance to be Little Miss Muffet and then the spider, as the rest of the class recites it. This activity will help the children practice taking turns and being a polite audience while others are dancing.

4. Bubble Gum: Recite this rhyme with the children: *Bubble gum, bubble gum, in a dish, how many pieces do you wish? 1, 2, 3, POP!* Now have the children stand in a personal space, and as you recite it again, prompt them to make a low shape with their bodies on count 1, a higher shape on count 2, and the highest shape they can on count 3. When you say "POP" they should fall to the floor.

Variation: Change the number of counts before the "POP."

Good-Bye Circle

Gather the children in a circle and recite this rhyme: *Head, shoulders, knees, arms high, everybody wave good-bye!* Ask the children to touch each part of the body as it is named.

Notes

What was successful about this lesson?

Which ideas could have worked better? How could they be improved?

What ideas were generated by the children during the lesson?

How would you enhance or expand this lesson in the future?

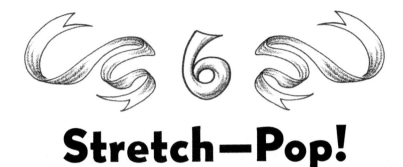

Stretch—Pop!

This lesson allows children to explore two qualities of movement: stretchy versus percussive. The contrast of these two movement qualities is a very clear example of how the use and flow of energy can change movement. The children will develop an increasing understanding of the different ways their own bodies can move. In addition, this lesson builds on the children's knowledge of opposites.

The children will also continue to practice using props responsibly, which will be a useful classroom management tool for you to have in later lessons.

MUSIC SUGGESTIONS:

General
It is helpful to have two distinct types of music for this lesson to reflect the qualities of the two types of movement that will be explored:

- For the "stretchy" movement: slow, flowing music
- For the "popping" movement: drums or percussion selections

Specific Selections
For the stretchy movement:

- "Lieder und Spielstucke: Andante" and "Zwei Taktwechseltanze" (*Orff-Schulwerk Vol. 1: Musica Poetica*, Carl Orff, Celestial Harmonies, 1995)

For the popping movement:

- "Funf Kleine Kanons" (*Orff-Schulwerk Vol. 1: Musica Poetica*, Carl Orff, Celestial Harmonies, 1995)
- "Pop Goes the Weasel!" (*Pop Goes the Weasel, A Silly Song Book*, Auerbach, Gaisey, Piggy Toes Press, 2005)
- "Popcorn Calling Me" (Laurie Berkner, *Buzz Buzz*, Two Tomatoes, 2001)

MATERIALS NEEDED:

- Soft stretchy fabric cut into strips about 12 inches long
- Drum

Early Learning Standards
11B, 17A

Opening Activity: Introduction to Stretching and Popping

1. Explore the Stretch: Seated in a circle with the students, ask, *What is one of the first things you do when you wake up in the morning? Do you know why you stretch? We stretch our bodies in the morning to get them ready to move. Can you think of some things that are stretchy?*

Now try moving around the room, stretching as if you are waking up your muscles. This helps our muscles get warmed up and ready to move!

2. Explore the Pop: Bring the children back to the circle and ask, *What happens if you stretch a rubber band too much? Can you think of other things that pop? Let's make popping sounds with our bodies.* Encourage the children to make noises with their mouths, clap or tap other parts of their bodies, jump and hop, etc.

3. Pop Goes the Weasel: If you have the music, play the song, and sing along with it. If you don't, recite or sing the words below once with the children. Repeat them, but this time have the children move in small circles in their personal spaces, pretending to circle a mulberry bush, and then fall to the floor on the word "pop!"

All around the mulberry bush
The monkey chased the weasel
The monkey thought it was all in fun
Pop! goes the weasel!

A penny for a spool of thread
A penny for the needle
That's the way the money goes
Pop! goes the weasel!

Teaching Tip: *Remind the children to catch themselves with their hands when falling quickly to the floor.*

Greeting Circle

Stand in a circle: *Let's make stretchy sounds with our voices as we go up and down to the floor. Then, as we go faster, we will make popping sounds.* Finish seated on the floor.

Movement Exploration

SEATED WARM-UPS

With the children seated on the floor in a circle, introduce the following warm-up exercises, which have reaches and bends:

1. Flex and Point Feet: *Can you flex and point your feet? Smile when your toes come toward you, and make a sad face when they point away from you. Let's try that again, but start out very slowly and get faster and faster! Now, use your feet to wave to different people around the circle.*

2. Upper Body Circles: Seated with legs crossed, curve the upper body to the side, continue moving until the torso is curved forward, and then to the other side, and back to the upright position, making a full circle. Then repeat to the other side.

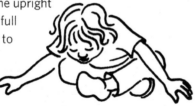

3. Pill Bug: With the children lying on the floor on their sides, prompt them to curl up and stretch out several times like a pill bug. Repeat, lying on the other side.

4. Bring the Children to Standing: Prompt each child to pretend to be a rubber band by lying on the floor. Ask them to slowly stretch themselves to standing, coming all the way to a tiptoe balance with their arms stretched high above their heads. When you clap your hands, the children fall quickly to the floor. Repeat several times.

FREE DANCES

Continue to explore the theme of stretch and pop with three very different free dances. The prop activity should generate many interesting movements. Take the opportunity to highlight students who solve the tasks with particular flair.

1. Free Dance about Stretchy Movement: Pass out the stretchy fabric strips, and play one of the Orff selections or other flowing music. Encourage the children to think of different ways of stretching the fabric and moving with a stretchy quality as they dance to the music.

 Teaching Tip: *Remind the class of guidelines for using props: The children should not touch another child with the prop. They should use the prop only as instructed: Hold on to it while dancing, and do not throw it or pull it in any way that could damage it. In addition, since these particular props are long strips of fabric, caution the children not to tie them in any way, and not to put them around their necks.*

Shine the Spotlight: Stop the class during the activity and ask the children to watch one student's creative idea as she stretches the fabric and moves in imaginative ways. Ask the class to pause for a moment: *Look at the way Ana can stretch her fabric while taking those giant steps across the floor. Let's all try that, and then try out other ways to move!* This technique is excellent for encouraging the other children to generate ideas, while bringing positive attention to the chosen student. Of course, it is important to make sure to call attention to different students, and try to distribute the praise evenly over the course of the classes. Use this technique often during different class activities.

When this exploration is finished, collect the fabric strips.

2. Free Dance about Popping Movement: Play the Orff selection, or other percussive music, such as "Popcorn Calling Me," for accompaniment, and encourage the children to move in sudden, accented bursts, like the percussion sounds in the music. Encourage them to add their own sounds to this dance.

3. Balloon Free Dance: To conclude the class, suggest one more dance that combines the ideas of stretch and pop: Ask the children to imagine they are a balloon, and to think about what color, shape, and size they would like to be. Tell them that you will count to five, and as you do, they will get very big, stretch, and fill up with air. Then they will imagine they are floating in the sky. You can play a flowing piece of music during this exercise. After a couple of minutes, explain that as you call each child's name one by one and clap your hands or beat the drum, he will pop and fall down.

Good-Bye Circle

Standing in a circle: *Let's first do a bow with a long, stretchy movement while making stretchy noises, and then let's do a bow making popping noises!*

Notes

What was successful about this lesson?

Which ideas could have worked better? How could they be improved?

What ideas were generated by the children during the lesson?

How would you enhance or expand this lesson in the future?

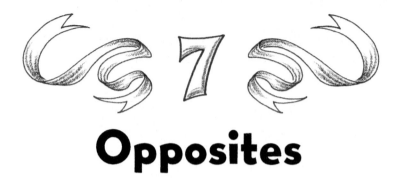

Opposites

This lesson uses movement to explore a myriad of opposites. The children will build on their knowledge of opposites from the last lesson, and then translate these concepts into movement. In addition, they will continue to explore how direction and energy affect their movements.

MUSIC SUGGESTIONS:

General
- A mix of different styles: classical, jazz, children's instrumentals, percussion, New Age, or electronic

Specific Selections
- *Orff-Schulwerk Vol. 1: Musica Poetica*, suggested for Lesson 6, also works well for this lesson
- "Vier Stucke für Xylophone" (from the Orff CD above) works well for the last activity of this lesson

MATERIALS NEEDED:
- *Understanding Opposites* (Playskool, Dutton Children's Books, 1997) or similar elementary book
- Drum

Early Learning Standards
11B, 12C

Opening Activity: Opposites

Begin this class by giving the children an initial lesson about opposites. Have the children stand in a personal space, and use the following sets of opposites with the accompanying directions:

1. High/Low: *Can you make yourself into a high shape? Now make yourself as low as you can.*

2. Straight/Curvy: *Can you make your body into a straight position, like uncooked spaghetti, and then a curvy one like wet noodles?*

> **Teaching Tip:** *Use concrete images whenever possible, such as "Make your body straight like uncooked spaghetti," or "curvy like a wet noodle!"*

3. Facing the Front of the Room/Facing the Back: *Face the front of the room, and then the back.*

4. Right Side Up/Upside Down: *You are standing right side up. How can you make yourself upside down?*

> **Teaching Tip:** *Use the spotlight technique of bringing attention to specific students who are solving the task creatively by stopping the class for brief demonstrations.*

Explain that these are all ideas of opposites. You can ask the class, *Do you remember that we danced about the opposites stretch and pop?*

Greeting Circle

Bring the children together into a circle. Tell them, *I am going to say hello very quietly, and I want you to say it back to me the same way. Then let's try the opposite of quiet. I will say it louder, and then you say it back to me the same way! Put your hands over your ears if you don't like loud noises!*

SEATED WARM-UP

While seated in a circle, introduce warm-ups that address opposites:

1. Body Part Isolations: Prompt the children to make faces and body gestures reflecting opposite emotions: happy vs. sad, calm vs. angry, scary vs. scared, silly vs. serious, excited vs. bored.

2. Wave: Wave "hello" and "good-bye" with different parts of the body.

3. Flex and Point Feet: Lead a flex and point exercise, and then ask the children to try it upside-down, lying on the back with the weight on the hands, and the feet raised one at a time in the air.

4. Merry-Go-Round: Seated with the knees close to the chest, use the arms to twirl yourself one way, and then the opposite way.

5. Boat: Seated with soles of feet together and knees apart, rock side to side in small waves, and then in giant waves.

MOTOR SKILLS PRACTICE

Line the children up across one end of the room with plenty of space in between them, and prompt them to go across the room together using these instructions: *Can you take little tiny baby steps all the way across the room? Now can you go across again trying the opposite, great big giant steps?* To elicit imaginative variations, try these other movement opposites: high/low, straight path/crooked path, forward/backward, cold floor/hot floor, smooth floor/sticky floor, slow/fast. Use any of the bands on the Orff CD that enhance the movement ideas.

EXPLORING MORE OPPOSITES

Gather the children together and read the book you brought about the concept of opposites. In the Playskool book, there are ideas for opposites that lend themselves well to movement, but it is not necessary to have the book. The opposites in the book are listed below.

Ask everyone to start out in a personal space in the room. Instrumental pieces such as "Vier Stucke fur Xylophone" are good accompaniments to this activity.

Explore the following opposites, calling them out one by one using the movement prompts:

1. Full/Empty: *Can you fill an imaginary container? Now empty it!*

2. Dirty/Clean: *Let's roll in the dirt! Now let's pretend we're in a giant washing machine—spinning 'round and 'round until we are clean!*

3. Open/Closed: *Can you open, and then close, a pretend door? Close it very quietly, and then pretend to slam it!*

4. Front/Back: *When I beat my drum, I want you to face the back of the room. Now face the front. Now try it again while I beat the drum faster!*

5. Little/Big: *Walk in a little circle around yourself. Now let's all come together in a big circle!*

6. In/Out: *Can you march into the corner of the room? Now march backward as you come out of the corner!*

7. Cold/Hot: *Let's pretend that the floor is so cold it is frozen, and we will skate on it! Now let's imagine that it turns into a hot road in the summer and we will run across it very quickly with our bare feet!*

Good-Bye Circle

In a circle, have the children bow toward the center of the circle, and then ask them, *How could we bow upside down?*

Notes

What was successful about this lesson?

Which ideas could have worked better? How could they be improved?

*What ideas were generated by the children during
the lesson?*

How would you enhance or expand this lesson in the future?

Part Two

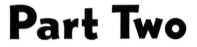

Lessons 8 through 38

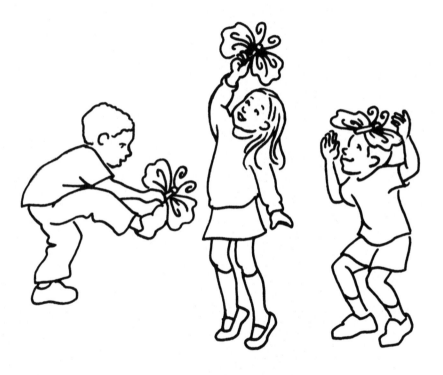

Applying Classroom Management Tools
and Building Basic Movement Skills

NOTE TO TEACHERS ABOUT PART TWO

The first seven lessons were presented in a step-by-step format, and you have now acquired the necessary tools for teaching the remaining classes. Part Two consists of thirty-one more themed lesson plans, and it is recommended that you proceed to this part once all of the lessons in the first part have been completed. However, if you already feel comfortable guiding the children in movement classes, proceed to this part at any time. You can return to the earlier lessons anytime you think that you or the children would benefit from the review, for reasons of maintaining order in the classroom, for reinforcement of any of the concepts, or simply to return to something more familiar. And, of course, you will continue to incorporate the techniques introduced in Part One as you teach the subsequent lessons.

The following Classroom Management Tools and Basic Movement Skills were introduced in Part One, and they will continue to be woven throughout the lessons in Part Two. All of the concepts below will be reinforced, expanded, and used in ways that will further stimulate and challenge the children in their exploration of movement:

CLASSROOM MANAGEMENT TOOLS

Listening to and Following Movement Instructions

Cues for Stopping

Personal Space and Shared Space

Guidelines for Free Group Movement

Group Cooperation and Taking Turns

Guidelines for Working with Props

Shine the Spotlight

BASIC MOVEMENT SKILLS

Control of Speed, or Tempo

Control of Direction in Space (includes level, direction, floor pattern, size)

Control of Energy (use of energy and flow to create a specific movement quality)

Body Awareness (includes body parts, balance, and shape)

Problem Solving through Movement

Locomotor Movements (moving from one place to another)

Moving with Rhythms, Music, or Sounds

Working with Props

Dramatic Play

Sequencing (learning a series of movements)

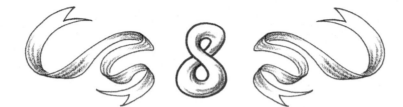

In the Harvest Meadow

This lesson is an imaginary trip to a meadow of tall grass in early autumn. The children will also be learning about the natural world as they explore the meadow and the animals that live there. Many of the lessons in this book are based on children's books or stories, which have endless amounts of imagination starters and movement images for dramatic play. This lesson is loosely based on the book *In the Tall, Tall Grass* by Denise Fleming, but it is not necessary to have the book.

MUSIC SUGGESTIONS:

General
- Music with nature sounds
- Music with a variety of tone and dynamic changes to represent different insects and animals

Specific Selections
- "Mother Earth's Routine" (*Mother Earth*, Tom Chapin, Gadfly, 2001)
- "The Wandering Piper" and "The Wind Dances" (*Celtic Awakening*, Howard Baer and Dan Gibson, 1997)
- *Echoes of Nature: The Natural Sounds of the Wilderness, Part 1* (Delta, 1993)

MATERIALS NEEDED:
- Optional: Small fiber-optic lights from a novelty store, or small flashlights
- Optional: The book *In the Tall, Tall Grass* by Denise Fleming (Henry Holt and Company, 1991), or pictures of animals that live in the meadow: caterpillars, hummingbirds, bees, ants, snakes, moles, beetles, frogs, rabbits, fireflies, and bats
- Drum

Early Learning Standards
4C, 12A, 12B

Opening Activity: Exploring the Meadow

Have the children begin in a personal space and suggest to the children that they pretend to be in a field before the cold autumn weather sets in. Prompt them with imagery such as tall grass to scramble through, little brooks to jump over, and small hills to climb. Play "Mother Earth's Routine," or another song or musical piece about nature, and prompt the children to play in the "meadow."

Greeting Circle

Bring the children together in a circle. Ask, *What other things might we find in a meadow in the early fall?*

Movement Exploration: The Harvest Meadow

SEATED WARM-UP

With the children seated in a circle, lead them in these warm-up exercises that incorporate the theme of the class.

1. Pill Bug: With the children lying on the floor on their sides, prompt them to curl up and stretch out several times like a pill bug. Repeat, lying on the other side.

2. Lizard Crawl: Lying face down, bend one leg up and to the side, and then use the arm and bent leg on that side to propel the body forward. Repeat to the other side, and continue moving forward by alternating sides.

3. Upside-Down Bug: *Have you ever seen a bug that is stuck on its back? Let's lie on the floor, and lift our legs and arms up toward the ceiling. Wave and bend your arms and legs slowly, and then faster and faster!*

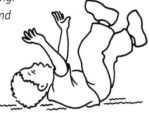

4. Bring the Children to Standing: *Jump up to standing, springing high like a grasshopper!*

MOTOR SKILLS PRACTICE

Line the children up on one side of the room, with plenty of space in between each child, and ask them to move across to the other side of the room according to each movement prompt. You will be expanding on the theme of the meadow during this activity, using the drum as accompaniment:

1. Walk: *Walk through a narrow path in the tall grass. First, let's follow a straight path. Then, as we go back to the other side of the room, let's make a crooked path!*

2. March: *Let's try to lift our knees higher than the grass!*

3. Tiptoe Walk: *Try to tiptoe very quietly, so we don't disturb the animals!*

4. Run: Introduce runs as a motor skill. Remind the children that running in a movement class is never a race. This helps to keep the children in control while they are running. The runs should be light and quick, always with bent-knee landings.

Ask the children to run slowly and heavily all together across the room, and then as lightly as possible ("hurry up and be quiet" runs) the next time. These light, quick runs are the proper technique for movement class. Remind the children to begin to slow down as they approach the other side of the room (*Put on your brakes!*). Once they have tried running several times, prompt them: *Imagine that you are running through the wind!*

DANCE STORY

1. Read the Book: Now gather the children together and either read the book, show pictures, or talk about animals in the tall grass. If you do not have access to the book, the order in which the animals appear is as follows: caterpillars, hummingbirds, bees, birds, ants, snakes, moles, beetles, frogs, rabbits, fireflies, and bats.

2. Dramatic Play: After reading the book or showing the pictures, ask the children to stand up and find a place to hide in the "grass." Play "The Wandering Piper," "The Wind Dances," or another soft background piece. Now read the book again slowly (or go through the pictures), and walk around showing the pages with pictures. As each new animal is introduced, ask the students how that animal moves, what color it is, what it eats, etc. Prompt them to move as each is named (*Let's be hummingbirds! Our wings are beating very fast!*).

Optional Props: For the fireflies and bats at the end of the story, turn out the lights (if this is possible, and if there are no obstructions in the space), and pass out the small fiber-optic lights or flashlights for the children to use as they dance. Repeat the cautions for the use of props: *Try not to touch another child with the prop, hold it carefully, and do not pull on it or throw it in a way that could damage it.*

Good-Bye Circle

Conclude the lesson sitting in a circle with the lights turned down, imagining you are in the meadow and watching the moon and stars in the clear night sky.

Notes

What was successful about this lesson?

Which ideas could have worked better? How could they be improved?

What ideas were generated by the children during the lesson?

How would you enhance or expand this lesson in the future?

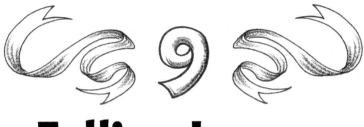

Falling Leaves

This class is a celebration of the autumn season. The children will dance about living things and explore the cycles of the seasons through movement. In addition, the children will be introduced to galloping as a large motor skill in this lesson.

MUSIC SUGGESTIONS:

General
- Upbeat music, such as bluegrass or a lively classical piece
- Calm, soothing music, such as environmental or New Age

Specific Selections
- "Shuckin' the Corn" and "Orange Blossom Special" (*Bluegrass Breakdown: 14 Instrumentals*, Easydisc, 1997), also used in Lesson 10
- "Autumn" (Vivaldi, *Vivaldi: Four Seasons*, Telarc, 1990)
- "Pocahontas" (Instrumental) (*Pocahontas: An Original Walt Disney Records Soundtrack*, Various Artists, Disney, 2001)

MATERIALS NEEDED:
- Pictures of nature in different seasons, and particularly pictures of fall colors
- Colorful leaves you have gathered, or pictures or cut-outs of leaves
- For the Quicksand game, masking tape or string if there are no lines or delineated areas in the classroom
- Drum

Early Learning Standards
12A, 12B, 12C

Opening Activity: Quicksand

1. Prepare the Space: For this game, you will need areas in the classroom that are "safe" and areas that are "quicksand." If there are any lines on the classroom floor, these can be incorporated into the game. Several parallel lines along the length of the floor work well, and they can be marked with masking tape or a thick string to make three or four long lines.

2. The Object of the Game: The children try to walk along the lines as if they are walking on tightropes, trying not to fall off. If they do fall off, they must crawl through the quicksand to another safe line. If the lines are close enough, the children can jump from one line to another. You can make up your own rules about passing if two children are on the same line and need to go by each other. For example, one or the other can back up, or one of the children must jump to another line.

3. Play the Game: Once the children understand the premise of the game, ask them to spread out along the lines to begin. Play a song from *Bluegrass Breakdown*, or another up-tempo piece, to start the game. The game will evolve based on the type of space you have, so be prepared for the children to be creative about the rules of this game!

Greeting Circle

Bring the children together into a circle and ask, *What are some of your favorite activities during the fall season?*

Movement Exploration: Falling Leaves

MOTOR SKILLS PRACTICE

Line the children up along one side of the room, and prompt them to practice the following large motor skills to the other side of the room, using autumn as a theme:

1. Walk: *Let's think about being outside on a warm fall day. What do you see as you are walking?*

2. Tiptoe Walk: *Can you try to tiptoe through crisp leaves and not make any noise?*

3. Run: *Imagine that you are running through a pile of leaves on the ground! Remember that these are "hurry up and be quiet" runs! Put on your brakes when you get close to the other side of the room.*

4. Gallop: Introduce gallops. Begin by beating the rhythm with a drum or tambourine: LOUD-quiet, LOUD-quiet, LOUD-quiet, GAL-lop, GAL-lop, GAL-lop. Ask the children to clap the rhythm, and then ask them to gallop across the floor while you are beating that rhythm, demonstrating if needed. The same foot leads throughout the gallop. Practicing the rhythm and repetition of the step is the best way for children to master gallops. Once the children have learned this motor skill, they should work toward galloping swiftly, in a controlled way, and quietly. *Gallop like a horse through the field!*

DANCE STORY

The next activity will be a movement improvisation, based on a story you will tell about a tree in changing seasons. The children will respond to the images and suggestions through movement.

1. Introduce the Activity: Have the children join you in a circle. Show the pictures and the leaves you have brought and talk about the changing seasons to prepare the children for the dance story. Ask them to find a personal space. Play the "Pocahontas" instrumental selection, or another calm, soothing piece, quietly as background music.

2. Begin the Story: *Imagine that you are a small seed, but you are the seed of a very large tree. You are deep in the rich soil under the ground in winter. Curl up like you are a seed.*

3. Spring: *It begins to get warm, and that is your signal to start to grow. Feel the sunlight and the rain, and stretch your roots deeply into the rich soil all around you. Slowly grow to be a strong, tall tree. Stand up now and reach toward the sky. You are beginning to sprout leaves! Look how you are changing!*

4. Summer: *Now it is summer! The sun is hot, and there are strong thunderstorms, with wind, lightning, and lots of hard rain. What does it feel like to have the warm sun, and then the cool rain, on your outstretched branches and waving leaves? What does it feel like when the wind whips through your leaves and branches, and moves you back and forth, up and down? See how the force of the wind can move your strong branches!*

5. Fall: *What happens in the fall? Imagine your leaves are turning red, orange, yellow, and brown. The leaves will begin to fall off of you, and when they do, they will swirl through the air.*

Now, let's pretend to be leaves! You are way up high and you are about to fall off the branches. Let go, and blow through the air, as you slowly fall to the ground. Play Vivaldi's "Autumn" or another upbeat selection during this part of the story. Elaborate on swirling, gliding, turning, and falling movements—this section can go on for a couple of minutes, so prompt the children to change the speed, level, and energy of their movements.

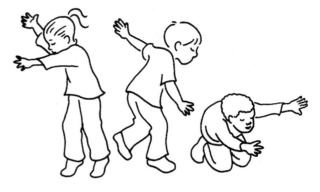

6. Conclude the Activity: *Let's each grab a rake, and rake up all of these leaves! We'll make a huge pile in the center of the room. Then we can line up and take turns jumping in the pile!* Have the children line up and, one at a time, take a running jump into the imaginary pile of leaves at the center of the room.

Good-Bye Circle

Bring the children together again. *Let's make a pretend campfire. We will gather some wood, and make a small fire. Because autumn nights are cold, let's warm our hands by the campfire.* Have the children sit down in a circle around the pretend campfire. *Now, let's curl up into our sleeping bags.* The following is a Native American song that you can recite softly to the children as they are imagining the autumn night:

> *Down the stream, down the stream, all the leaves go*
> *Down the stream, down the stream, all the leaves go*
> *Who can tell, who can know, where the leaves go?*
> *Who can tell, who can know, where the leaves go?*

Notes

What was successful about this lesson?

Which ideas could have worked better? How could they be improved?

What ideas were generated by the children during the lesson?

How would you enhance or expand this lesson in the future?

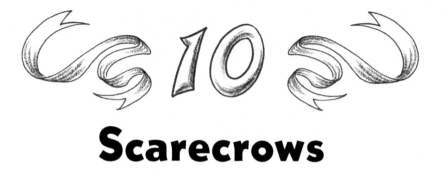

Scarecrows

Children will explore scarecrows through movement, and then will design and dance with their own scarecrow masks. In this lesson, the children learn to use a variety of different media to express themselves.

MUSIC SUGGESTIONS:

General
• Upbeat instrumental pieces, such as bluegrass or country

Specific Selection
• "Shuckin' the Corn" and "Orange Blossom Special" or other selections (*Bluegrass Breakdown: 14 Instrumentals*, Easydisc, 1997), as used in the previous lesson

MATERIALS NEEDED:
• Plain white paper plates, into which you have cut large holes for eyes
• Yarn (stapled or glued to the plates for hair)
• Crayons
• A book about scarecrows, especially one with lots of pictures. Some suggestions: *Scarecrows* (Lola M. Schaefer, Capstone Press, 1999); *Hello Mr. Scarecrow* (Rob Lewis, Farrar, Straus & Giroux, 1988); *Scarecrow* (Cynthia Rylant, Sagebrush Bound, 2001); *The Scarecrow's Hat* (Ken Brown, Peachtree Publishers, 2001); *Barn Dance* (Bill Martin, Jr., and John Archambault, Henry Holt & Co., 1988). If you don't have a book, find or draw pictures of several different scarecrows.
• Drum

Early Learning Standards
4C, 14A, 16B

Opening Activity: Mice and Crows

1. Introduce the Poem: Begin this class by reciting this version of a short nursery rhyme:

> One for the mouse
> One for the crow
> One to stop
> One to go.

2. Recite the Poem Together: Repeat the poem several times, asking the children to recite it with you. Explain to the children what a crow is, if they are unfamiliar with this word.

3. Respond with Movement: Instruct the children to begin in a personal space in the room. Tell them that you are going to say the poem again, and when you say the word *mouse*, they will go down to the ground, and when you say *crow*, they will go up on their tiptoes and reach their arms high. When you say *stop*, they freeze, and when you say *go*, they move around the room in a controlled way. Allow the children a short time to move on the word "go," and then beat the drum as a stop signal. Repeat this activity several times.

Greeting Circle

Have you ever seen a scarecrow? Where do you usually see them? Do you know why scarecrows are used, and how they can help farmers?

Movement Exploration: Scarecrows

MOTOR SKILLS PRACTICE

Line the children up on one end of the room and have them practice these large motor skills incorporating the lesson theme as they move together to the other side of the room:

1. Walk: *Let's follow a winding path through a cornfield!*

2. March: *March like a stiff scarecrow, swinging your arms at your sides!*

3. Tiptoe Walk: *Let's sneak through the forest!*

4. Gallop: *Gallop through the leaves!*

5. Slide: Introduce this motor skill, which is a sideways gallop. As with gallops, try beating the rhythm first so the children understand the rhythm of the movement, and then demonstrate the slides yourself, and finally, have the children try the movement. The rhythm of a slide, like a gallop, is LOUD-quiet, LOUD-quiet, LOUD-quiet, SLIDE-and, SLIDE-and, SLIDE-and. The same foot is always the lead foot in a slide, and the body faces and travels sideways. In the loud beat, the body is airborne and the following leg briefly taps or comes toward the leading leg in the air, and then lands first with a soft knee-bend.

Once they begin to master this skill, try slides while facing a partner. Pair up the children, place them in a line along one end of the room, and if there is an extra child, partner with her. Each child should face her partner, not holding hands, but stretching arms out to the side, as if holding a large circle between them. Once the children are all paired up in this ready position, beat the rhythm of the slide, and let them go together across the floor: *Pretend to hold a giant pumpkin between you and your partner!*

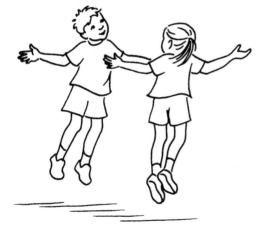

6. Run: *Can you run quickly and quietly? Now can you run like a floppy scarecrow?*

DANCE STORY

1. Read the Scarecrow Book: Gather the children together, and read the book you brought or show the pictures of scarecrows. Then lead a discussion by asking the children what kinds of scarecrows they saw in the book, and what kind of scarecrow they would each like to imagine they could be.

2. Try Moving Like a Scarecrow: Talk about how a scarecrow would move: *If he had strong sticks holding him up, he would move in a straight and stiff way, but if you took him off of the sticks, he would be very floppy.* With the bluegrass or country music playing, prompt them to try the different movement qualities (stiff, then floppy).

3. Make Masks: Now pass out the paper plates that have eye holes and glued or stapled yarn for hair. Give each of the children a few crayons, and let them draw their own scarecrow face, reminding them that they can be happy, sad, funny, or any kind of scarecrow they wish to be.

4. Dance with the Masks: Now ask the children to move holding their scarecrow masks to their faces or in their hands. Prompt them to dance about the floppy and stiff scarecrows, as well as about the emotions in the faces they have drawn. Encourage them to dance about ideas they get from the other children's masks as well.

> *Teaching Tip:* These scarecrow dances are a good opportunity for the teacher to pause occasionally and shine the spotlight on a specific child's approach to the movement tasks. In addition to the positive reinforcement, this technique inspires movement ideas in the other children.

Good-Bye Circle

Bow like a stiff scarecrow, and then like a floppy one!

Notes

What was successful about this lesson?

*Which ideas could have worked better? How could they
be improved?*

*What ideas were generated by the children during
the lesson?*

How would you enhance or expand this lesson in the future?

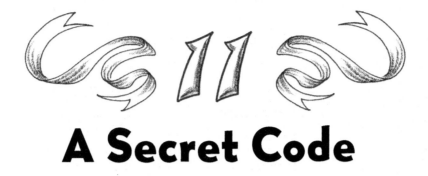

A Secret Code

This lesson, and its companion, Lesson 12: A Secret Map, is a way for young children to learn and perform movements through the use of symbols. In this lesson, the children will learn to understand, copy, and translate printed symbols into particular movements. These skills lay an important groundwork for early reading. By the end of this class, the child will respond to the symbols with movement.

MUSIC SUGGESTIONS:

General
- A long track of soft background music, such as New Age

Specific Selection
- *Autumn*, George Winston (Windham Hill Records, 2001)

MATERIALS NEEDED
- Movement Code Chart (explained below)
- File cards, each with one symbol drawn as large as possible, which will be your Secret Code Cards
- Large roll of paper, like a roll of butcher paper
- Crayons or markers (a variety of colors)

Early Learning Standards
6A, 10B, 11D

This lesson and its companion, Lesson 12, are structured differently than most of the lessons in this book. The four sections of the Lesson Description are woven together rather than listed separately.

1. Prepare the Secret Code: Below is the "Secret Code," or Movement Code. Make a chart of the code on a large posterboard. It is not necessary to write what each symbol represents on the posterboard. You will be going over that information later with the children. Then write each symbol on an index card.

MOVEMENT CODE

!	Starting or Ending Position
X	Stop
- - - -	Walk
. . . .	Run
II	Jump
I	Hop
O	Turn

2. Introduction of the Movement Code: Gather the children together, and ask them if they know what a secret code is. Explain to them that this class will be a chance for them to learn a secret code.

Next, show the index cards of the code one by one. Explain each one, and then go through them a few more times so that the children can become visually familiar with the symbols.

3. Learning the Symbols: Take the file cards and put them in the following order, which begins with the easier movements, and works up to the larger motor skills: **!, - - - -, X, O, II, I, ...**

Ask the children to find a beginning position in a personal space in the room by showing the **!** symbol. The children can begin in any position they like, as long as they know that this is the symbol for the starting position.

Then show them the **- - - -** symbol, and instruct them to walk around the room. Prompt them to think of variations on a plain walk: *Can you walk in different directions? Can you walk very high, and then very low?* Interject the **X** symbol periodically during the walks, so that they can learn the stop cue for this lesson.

Show the **O**, or turning symbol. As the children continue walking, ask them to add turns: *Let's see how many different ways we can turn. Can you turn to get yourself to the floor? Can you turn around while you are on the floor? How can you turn to get yourself back up to standing?*

Next, try the **II** (two-footed jumping) symbol. Ask the children: *Can you jump in place? Can you jump while turning? Can you jump around the room?* Try the same prompts with the **I** (one-footed hopping) symbol. Show the **. . . .** symbol, and prompt the children to run in a controlled way around the room. Once the children have become familiar with all of the symbols, show the **!** once again, for a final position.

At this point in the lesson, three important things have been accomplished. First, the students have had a thorough warm-up. Second, they have become visually familiar with the symbols that they will use in the code, and third, they can translate the symbols into movement.

Teaching Tip: *If you want to teach this lesson in two sessions, this is a good stopping point. Start the next lesson with a brief review of the Learning the Symbols activity, and then proceed to Writing the Symbols.*

4. Writing the Symbols: Unroll a long sheet of paper in the middle of the room, and pass out the crayons or markers. Ask the children to sit around the edges of the paper. Put on some soothing background music, such as a quiet selection from *Autumn* by George Winston. Ask the children to write each symbol down one by one, as you remind them what the symbols represent, and let them practice writing each symbol several times.

5. Reinforcing the Learning of the Symbols: Once they have shown that they can write all or at least some of the symbols, clear the paper and markers. Ask each child to find a personal space in the room and think of a starting position. Put on a selection of music that is more lively, such as an upbeat track from the same CD. Using the index cards again, randomly show the symbols to the children, and prompt them to respond with the appropriate movements. Go through the cards more than once, mixing them up so that they are in a different order each time.

6. Conclude the Lesson: *In our next movement class, you will learn to make a secret map using the secret code!*

LESSON SUPPLEMENT

The movement code can be expanded for older children, or for further exploration of the symbol concepts. Below are ideas for more symbols to use in extending the lesson, which may become one or several more lessons. In addition, the children may want to make up their own symbols.

↓	Go down to the floor
↑	Come up from the floor
☺	Make a face
ɯ	Skips
∧	One big traveling jump or leap
✷	Surprise (make up a movement)
→	Go forward
←	Go backward

Notes

What was successful about this lesson?

Which ideas could have worked better? How could they be improved?

What ideas were generated by the children during the lesson?

How would you enhance or expand this lesson in the future?

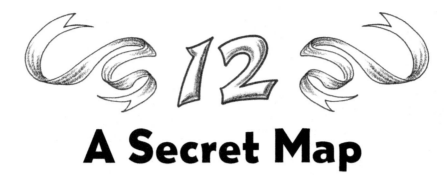

A Secret Map

This lesson is a continuation of Lesson 11, and is a further refinement of the movement code. The children will begin to create their own dance sequences, using the symbols as a kind of map. Making a movement map helps children understand that written symbols can have meaning, which is an important skill for learning to read and write.

MUSIC SUGGESTIONS:

General
- Two or three different instrumental pieces that are upbeat and fun, but with different qualities (tempo, rhythm, or style of music)

Specific Selections
- "Gallop" (*Classics for Kids*, RCA, 1993)
- "Palm Leaf Rag" (Coleman, Joplin, *The Complete Rags of Scott Joplin*, Music Masters Jazz, 1995)
- A children's song that is a class favorite

MATERIALS NEEDED:
- Movement Code Chart (from Lesson 11)
- Secret Code Cards (from Lesson 11)
- White or colored 8½ x 11 inch paper
- Crayons or markers (a variety of colors)
- Optional: Examples of treasure maps

Early Learning Standards
6A, 10B, 11D

As in Lesson 11, this lesson is structured differently than the others in this book. The four sections of the Lesson Description are interwoven rather than listed separately.

1. Review the Movement Code: Begin this class with a review of the movement code from the last lesson, using the Secret Code Cards. Stand in the middle of the room, with the children spread out in their own personal spaces. Hold up a card, and ask the children what the card represents. Encourage them to try the movement, but ask them to move only in their personal spaces, so that they walk, jump, hop, turn, and run in place. This exercise will also serve as an effective warm-up.

2. Bring Them to the Greeting Circle: To bring the children into the Greeting Circle, call out their names one by one. As you call out each name, also switch to a new card, and have the child use that movement to get to the center of the room.

For the **X** (stop) symbol, which isn't a traveling movement, help the child use his imagination, such as *Take three steps and stop (repeat as needed) until you get to the center!* For the **!** symbol, suggest, *Can you make a shape, and then travel in that shape to the center of the room?*

After each child has had a chance to perform a movement from the Secret Code Cards to the center of the room, sit down in a circle with the children.

3. Greeting Circle—Introducing the Map Idea: *Have you ever heard of a treasure map? A treasure map tells people where to go and how to get there, so they can find what they are looking for.* If you have brought any examples of treasure maps, show them to the children.

We are going to make our own maps that will also tell us where to go and how to move using the movement code we have learned.

4. Using the Secret Code to Make a Map: Give each child a sheet of paper, and pass out the crayons or markers. Hold up the Movement Code Chart. Ask the children to think of a starting position, and draw a **!**, which will symbolize the beginnings of their dances.

Then ask them to choose and draw three to five movement symbols. For each symbol, have them draw how many of that movement they would like to do. For example, **O O O**, would be three turns in a row. The map ends with another **!**, which will be the ending position of the movement phrase they are creating. The children can write the symbols in a line, or in a column, or however they choose to set it up.

5. Following the Map: Once the children have finished drawing their movement maps, ask them to take the map and, walking, try to follow the map and learn the movements in order. The children should mark (indicate with less energetic movement) the movements, because they will be looking at their maps and not watching carefully where they are going. If the class is very large, it is best to divide the class into smaller groups for this part, and have the other children watch as each group learns its maps.

6. Trying the Movement Without the Map: Once the children have learned their movement maps, have them put their maps down in a place away from the dancing area. In small groups, ask them if they can remember what their secret maps tell them to do. Ask them to practice their movement sequences a few times from memory.

    Important Note: If the children don't remember their movements and want to continue to use their maps, that is fine. It would be helpful, though, to encourage them to try their phrases without the maps at least once by the end of the lesson. The important thing is not that they remember their movement exactly, but that they understand that making a movement map has helped them to create a movement sequence and that writing has meaning. If the dance has changed from the exact steps of the map, that is okay—in fact, it might even be better than what they envisioned when they wrote their sequence of movement using the code. As has been stated many times, if the children are engaged and moving, they are learning.

7. Performing the Movement with Music: Now they are ready to perform their dance phrases with music. For this, it is good to have the children work in small groups of four or five, and have the rest of the class be the audience. Try different kinds of music, and let each group dance to a selection. They will probably have a favorite selection, so let them try their dances one last time at the end of class to the consensus favorite, performing their movement sequences all

together if there is room, or again in small groups if this works better. Remind the children to try to stay within their bubbles of space.

8. Conclude the Lesson: Allow the children to take their maps home, and tell them that they will have to explain to other people the meaning of their secret maps, because they are the only ones who know how to read the secret code!

Variation: Children often like to draw a new movement map once they are more familiar with the symbols. In that case, repeat the sections Following the Map, Trying the Movement Without the Map, and Performing the Movement with Music with these new maps. In addition, expand the possibilities for new ideas by using the supplementary symbols listed at the end of Lesson 11, or encourage the children to make up their own symbols.

Notes

What was successful about this lesson?

Which ideas could have worked better? How could they be improved?

What ideas were generated by the children during the lesson?

How would you enhance or expand this lesson in the future?

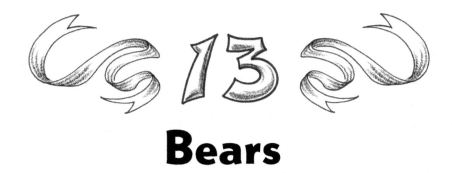

Bears

In this lesson, the children will use bears as inspiration for creative movement. In doing so, they will expand their knowledge of the natural world, learning about different types of bears, the many ways bears move, and the concept of hibernation.

MUSIC SUGGESTIONS:

General

- One flowing background instrumental, such as New Age or environmental
- One upbeat instrumental or song, preferably about bears

Specific Selections

- "On the Day You Were Born" (instrumental) (*On the Day You Were Born*, Debra Frasier, composed by Matthew Smith, Harcourt Children's Books, 2005) (hardcover and musical CD edition)
- "The Bear Cha-Cha-Cha" (*Songs from Jim Henson's Bear in the Big Blue House*, Various Artists, Disney, 2000)

MATERIALS NEEDED:

- A book, or collection of illustrations or photos, of different kinds of bears
- A large cloth (about 6 x 6 feet), preferably black or another dark color
- Drum

Early Learning Standards
12A, 12B

Opening Activity: Teddy Bears

Begin this class by reciting this short version of the poem "Teddy Bear":

Teddy bear, teddy bear	*Teddy bear, teddy bear*
Turn around	*Dance on your toes*
Teddy bear, teddy bear	*Teddy bear, teddy bear*
Touch the ground	*Touch your nose*

Repeat until the children learn the words, and then encourage them to recite and perform the movements at the same time.

Greeting Circle

Bring the children together in a circle. Tell them, *Today we are going to dance about bears—how many kinds can we think of? Do you know what hibernation is? In the fall, bears eat lots and lots of food to store up for the winter. Then they sleep for the whole winter and wake up when it's warm again in the spring!*

Movement Exploration: A Big Black Bear

SEATED WARM-UP

With the children still seated in a circle, begin with a warm-up exercise that addresses the lesson theme:

Body Part Isolations: *Let's imagine we are bears, and try out our different body parts. Can you open and close your bear eyes? Your mouth? What would it be* *like to have big bear ears—let's imagine we could wiggle them! Move your strong bear arms, your legs, your big bear paws!*

MOTOR SKILLS PRACTICE

Now have the children line up on one side of the classroom. Have the children practice these large motor skills, moving across the floor from one end of the room to the other and using the lesson theme for prompts:

1. Walk: *How would a baby bear walk? How would it be different from the way a great big bear would walk?*

2. March: *Let's make a bear parade!*

3. Gallop: *Let's see how fast bears can gallop!*

4. Slide: *Face your partner, and hold your bear arms wide. Can you stay facing your partner, close but not touching, all the way across the room?*

5. Run: *How fast can bears run, still being in control, and putting on their brakes so they can stop when they get to the other side of the room?*

6. Jump: *Let's try doing four big jumps, and then land in a bear shape!* This exercise can be done in place, after practicing the traveling skills.

Variation: Ask the children to think of all the other things bears can do: Pandas climb, polar bears swim, bear cubs love to roll and play, and many kinds of bears wade in the water to fish. Prompt them with these ideas, and ask them to think of their own.

DANCE STORY

1. Prepare the Activity: Ask the children to go to a personal space. Have your large black cloth handy and play the instrumental music "On the Day You Were Born" or another quiet piece for background music.

2. Narrate the Story: Narrate the following story:

Imagine that you are a big black bear. First, you look for food, because winter is almost here, and you need to store up lots of body fat to get you through the long winter. Reach high for those berries and nuts! Search for food all around the room. Now you have to find the perfect cave in which to spend the winter. Where will you find one?

Look—here is a large, dark cave! Hold up the black cloth. Let the children come underneath. *You are hibernating. Do you remember what that means? You are sleeping through the whole winter!*

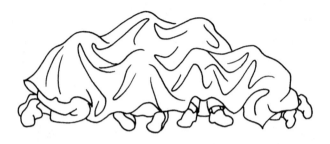

To encourage the children to wait a short time under the cloth, ask questions about the cave: *What shape would you be when you are all curled up? What shape is the cave? Is it nice and warm in the cave? Can you hear the sound of your own breath? Can you slow down your breathing, like a hibernating bear?* Wait a short time before beginning the next section of the story.

Can you imagine how hard it would be to wake up after that long sleep? Now it is spring! Peek out of the cloth and look at the beautiful, sunny day. Blink your eyes to get them used to the light. Stand up slowly, yawn, and stretch, like you stretch in the morning after sleeping all night. Aren't you hungry after all that time with no food?

Hurry and look for food again, and enjoy the feeling of moving after that long winter in the cave. Run and play and enjoy the warm spring day! Once they have all emerged from the cloth, change the music to "The Bear Cha-Cha-Cha" or another upbeat musical piece for this last part of the dance story.

Good-Bye Circle

Bring the children together again and ask, *How would a bear bow?*

Notes

What was successful about this lesson?

Which ideas could have worked better? How could they be improved?

What ideas were generated by the children during the lesson?

How would you enhance or expand this lesson in the future?

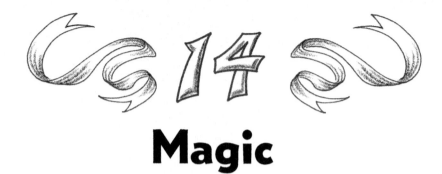

Magic

The children will use movement games as an entryway to an imaginary enchanted world. Creativity and imagination are valuable skills for children to develop in early childhood.

MUSIC SUGGESTIONS:

General

- Music that is reminiscent of merry-go-rounds, music boxes, or magical settings, such as harpsichord, bells, harp, or calliope

Specific Selections

- "Golden Dream" (*Ragtime at the Magical Kingdoms*, Chris Calabrese, Siren, 1998)
- "Carousel Dreams" or other selections (*Circus Clown Calliope, Vols. 1 & 2*, Various Artists, The Orchard, 1999)
- "The Bells Go Ringing" or other selections (*Victorian Music Boxes*, Various Artists, Saydisc, 1995)

MATERIALS NEEDED:

- A wand (handmade or from a costume store)
- The book *Up and Down on the Merry-Go-Round* (Bill Martin, Jr. & John Archambault, Henry Holt and Company, 1985 and 1988), or another book or pictures of a merry-go-round
- Drum (preferably a Djembe drum)

Early Learning Standards
4C, 16B, 22C

Opening Activity: The Magician and the Magic Drum

1. Have the children stand in a circle as you present the idea of an imaginary magician using his powers to help the children dance:
First the magician tells us to move our toes, and only

our toes, and then our elbows. Now we can only move our eyes. . . . *As you name each body part, explore its range of movement while beating the drum, so that a warm-up is accomplished through isolation exercises.

2. Now we will move our whole bodies. If you have a Djembe drum, say the following: *I will use my Djembe drum to keep the beat as we move. Did you know that the Djembe drum is a special African drum, and drum masters there call it a magic drum because it has the power to make people dance?* Play the piece "Golden Dream" or another dreamy, magical selection, and allow the children to move freely, now that they have warmed up the different parts of the body.

Greeting Circle

Have you ever wished you had a magic wand? What would you use your magic wand to do? We are going to dance about magic!

Movement Exploration

MOTOR SKILLS PRACTICE

Moving together from one end of the room to the other, practice these motor skills using magical images. Remind the children to move in their personal bubbles of space:

1. Walk *like an enchanted king or queen.*

2. March *like a soldier guarding a magical castle.*

3. Tiptoe Walk *so quietly you could pretend you were invisible.*

4. Gallop *like a unicorn.*

5. Jump: *Let's jump to the beat of the Djembe* (or any drum). *Try eight jumps in place, and then eight jumps moving around the room!*

MERRY-GO-ROUND DANCE

1. Read the Book: Gather the children together and read the book or show the pictures you have brought about a merry-go-round.

2. Merry-Go-Round Dance: Stand in a large circle with the children. Take out the "magic wand" you have brought, and tell them that with the wand you are going to pretend to turn them all into merry-go-round animals. Prompt their imaginations with questions: *What kind of merry-go-round animal would you like to be? What color is your animal?* Wave the wand over the children. Play "Carousel Dreams," or another magical-sounding musical selection, and have the children move in a circle, pretending they are on a merry-go-round.

While they are moving, encourage the children to try using different steps and different body shapes. Prompt them with questions such as *How does your animal move as it goes around the merry-go-round? Does it go up and down and around at the same time?* They might want to change into different animals several times during this improvisation, so wave your wand over them when they want to try a new animal idea.

3. Magic Wand Dance: Tell the children that they will now leave the merry-go-round and enter the magical world around them. Ask each child, *What would you like to be?* Prompt them with ideas if necessary, such as, *Do you have a favorite character from a book you would like to dance about? Would you like to imagine you can fly?* Tap each child on the shoulder with the wand and let them all dance about their specific ideas. If they want to change ideas during the game, encourage them to come up for another tap on the shoulder whenever they want to try out a new idea. Good accompaniment for this activity is "The Bells Go Ringing" or other music that is reminiscent of a magical setting.

Variation: If there is time, give each child a turn to hold the wand and be the "magician" for the other children.

Good-Bye Circle

Gather the children back into a circle and "change" them back into children by waving the wand over them.

Notes

What was successful about this lesson?

Which ideas could have worked better? How could they be improved?

What ideas were generated by the children during the lesson?

How would you enhance or expand this lesson in the future?

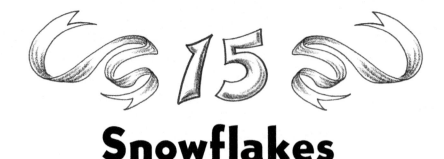

Snowflakes

The many aspects of snow and snowflakes provide ideas for imaginative movement activities in this lesson. Children will have the opportunity to explore the different characteristics of the winter season, expanding their knowledge and appreciation of the natural world. In addition, the children will continue to practice moving with props.

MUSIC SUGGESTIONS:

General
- Upbeat instrumental music, especially light classical pieces, as well as any songs about winter

Specific Selections
- "Cozy Bug Twist" (*Dance in Your Pants*, David Jack, Ta-Dum Productions, 2002)
- "Blue Danube Waltz" (*Mad about Cartoons*, Various Artists, Deutsche Grammophon, 1993)
- "Winter" (*Vivaldi: The Four Seasons*, Telarc, 1990)

MATERIALS NEEDED:
- "Snowflakes," which you have made out of white tulle netting: cut strips about 6 inches wide and about 9 inches long. Tie two of them together with a knot in the center, and fluff out the four sides to make the snowflakes. The tulle netting is sold by the yard or in ribbon spools at fabric stores; it is very inexpensive and easy to use
- Drum

Early Learning Standards
12A, 16A

Opening Activity

In this activity, the children will be exploring different ways of making twisty shapes with their bodies.

Move and Freeze in Twisty Shapes: Start by playing a winter-themed song like "Cozy Bug Twist" or an upbeat instrumental selection. Let the children dance freely to the music. Then stop the music occasionally, and call out, *Freeze in a twisty shape like a pretzel!* Prompt them with the following ideas that evoke twisty shapes, many of which involve images of winter: a bear curled up for a winter nap, a braid, a pretzel, hugging yourself to keep warm, curling up under a warm blanket, a barbershop pole, steam rising up from a cup of hot chocolate, an ice-skater making figure-eight patterns, a kitten tangling up a ball of yarn.

Greeting Circle

What is your favorite winter activity?

Movement Exploration

SEATED WARM-UP

Lead the children through the following warm-ups seated in a circle, adapting them to fit the winter theme.

1. Boat: In this lesson, the boat is now a sled. Seated with soles of feet together and knees apart, rock side to side as if sitting on a sled going down a hill. On different counts, have the children "fall off the sled" by falling to the floor.

2. Merry-Go-Round: Seated with knees close to chest, use arms to twirl yourself around. Use the idea of turning around on a saucer sled instead of a merry-go-round.

3. Snow Wings: Lie on the ground facing the ceiling, and move arms and legs, as if to make a winged shape in the snow.

4. Bring the Children to Standing: Suggest that the children each roll a big snowball, and then stand up and try to pick up the large, heavy snowball. Then ask the children to throw their big snowball up in the air and catch it, or to pretend to throw it to someone else.

MOTOR SKILLS PRACTICE

Moving across the floor from one end of the room to the other, practice these large motor skills all together using the lesson theme for prompts:

1. Slide: Line the children up in pairs on one side of the room. Prompt each pair to pretend to hold a great big snowball between them (not holding hands, but maintaining their face-to-face position). *Slide across the floor, and don't drop your snowball!*

2. Lunge: *We are going to do a very different kind of walking. It is a giant step! We reach our legs very far when we do a lunge.* Show a lunge, taking a large step while bending the front knee. Instruct the children to try several in a row, alternating each one, showing that it is a walk with giant steps. *Pretend we are walking through very deep snow!*

SNOWFLAKE DANCE

1. Introduce the Dance: This activity is a free dance improvisation about snowflakes. Begin by asking the students to think about snowflakes: *Are they all the same? Are some bigger than others? Are they light or heavy? If you were a snowflake, what would you look like?*

Put on some lively music, such as the "Blue Danube Waltz," and ask them to move like a snowflake. While they are dancing, suggest other winter-inspired movement ideas, such as swirling like the wind, becoming a heavy, wet snowflake, and jumping over a snowbank.

2. Snowflake Dance with Props: Pass out the tulle snowflakes. Play "Winter: Allegro," or a similar selection, and prompt the children to move with their props. Encourage them to continue to dance about the different qualities of snowflakes (light, heavy, blowing, falling, swirling) as well as to have fun with the prop. For example: *Let's try to make a snowstorm by throwing our snowflakes up in the air at the same time!*

Teaching Tip: Remind the children of the guidelines for using props. The children should not touch another child with the prop. They should use the prop only as instructed, holding on to it while dancing, and making sure not to pull on it in a way that could damage it.

Good-Bye Circle

Use the prop for the final bow, having the children hold the snowflake in one hand, and bow with a flourish by bringing that hand forward across the body during the bow.

Notes

What was successful about this lesson?

Which ideas could have worked better? How could they be improved?

What ideas were generated by the children during the lesson?

How would you enhance or expand this lesson in the future?

16

What Is This and How Does It Move?

This lesson uses everyday objects to demonstrate the idea of "how" something moves. The "how" is called movement quality, which is the use of energy and flow. By looking at different objects and observing how they each move, the children will be learning to see patterns in objects that are seemingly different based on a single characteristic, in this case, movement. The children will also have the chance to build on their vocabularies as you call out different ways of moving.

MUSIC SUGGESTIONS:

General
- One or two selections that would serve as quiet background music, such as environmental or New Age music
- One lively, upbeat song or instrumental

Specific Selections
- "Kalimba Suite" (*Beyond Words*, Bobby McFerrin, Blue Note Records, 2002)
- "On the Day You Were Born" (instrumental) (*On the Day You Were Born*, Debra Frasier, composed by Matthew Smith, Harcourt Children's Books, 2005) (hardcover and musical CD edition)
- "Dancin' Machine" (Greg & Steve, *We All Live Together Vol. 3*, Youngheart, 1998)

MATERIALS NEEDED:
- Bag of Found Objects: In a brightly colored paper or cloth bag, place eight or ten small items you have collected that evoke movement, such as: a top, a plastic grasshopper, a Koosh® ball, a candle, a stretchy band, a spring, a pipe cleaner, a feather, a small bouncy ball, a snow globe, a scarf, a balloon, a stick with Mylar® streamers, and anything else that you have readily available.
- Drum

Early Learning Standards
1C, 10C, 11B

Opening Activity

The class will begin with a free dance in which you call out different action words. Many of the words you will use for this activity come from the Effort-Shape theory of movement dynamics, which studies how the use of different energy affects the way a person moves. Each word evokes a specific quality: JIGGLE, COLLAPSE, SWING, DAB, MELT, STOMP, TWIRL, SNEAK, BOUNCE, SLINK, CROUCH, DART, STRETCH, SOAR, TRUDGE, FLOP. You can add any more that you wish.

Teacher's Tip: While teaching movement to young children, keep in mind that using concrete cues and prompts in your instructions is very helpful. Many descriptive movement words, such as "crouch" or "twirl," are more readily understood by children with the simple addition of an image, such as "crouch like a cat" or "twirl like a top." As some of the words may be unfamiliar to the children, be prepared to demonstrate.

1. Action Word Dance: Play a track of music that will lend itself to many kinds of movement, such as "Kalimba Suite," as a background to this activity. Instruct the children to begin to move freely to the music. Then begin to call out the different actions one by one, giving examples such as, *Can you jiggle like a washing machine? Now can you melt like a candle? Can* you pretend to dab paint onto the air with your finger? Your foot? Your head? Can you trudge through a muddy swamp? Can you bounce like you are on a trampoline?

2. Stopping: At the end of the exercise, try different kinds of stopping: *Can you stop slowly like a big train putting on its brakes? Can you stop suddenly? Can you stop and collapse in slow motion? Can you stop and flop quickly onto the floor?*

Greeting Circle

1. Gather the children together in a circle and ask, *Did you notice how we used different amounts of energy in that last exercise?*

2. *Now try going from sitting to standing, the way you usually do it. That doesn't take too much energy, does it? Sit down, and we will try another way of standing up. Imagine you are holding a very heavy rock, and you have to go from sitting to standing. You have to use more energy, and it changes the way you move when you are trying to stand up! Do you see how the way we use energy affects our movement? We will try out many different ways to use energy in this lesson, and we will see how our movement changes.*

Movement Exploration

SEATED WARM-UPS

Lead the following seated warm-ups, using descriptive words as you did in the opening activity. In these warm-ups, the children will continue to explore how the use of energy affects movement:

1. Boat: Seated with the soles of the feet together, rock back and forth. Use phrases such as *jiggle like a motor boat, bounce through waves,* or *soar like a sailboat!*

2. Kitty-Cat: *On hands and knees, curve and arch your back like a lazy cat and then a very frisky, playful cat.*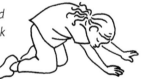

3. Snow Wings: Lying on the ground, move arms and legs, as if to make a winged shape in the snow. *Make soft, slow small wings and then big, sweeping wing strokes!*

MOTOR SKILLS PRACTICE

Continue the theme of movement quality as you lead the children through the following large motor skills. Have the children line up on one side of the room and practice these skills together to the other side:

1. Walk: *Let's walk like we are slowly collapsing, and then waddle back across like a duck.*

2. Tiptoe Walk: *Let's do our tiptoe walks first like we are stretching as high as we can. Now let's tiptoe back to the other side like we are sneaking.*

3. March: *Let's march like we are stomping, and then very lightly without making any noise.*

4. Run: *Can you run quickly and lightly, and then imagine you are trying to run through a room filled up with water?*

FOUND OBJECTS

1. Prepare the Activity: Now you will bring out your bag of found objects. Stand at the front of the room, and have the children begin in a personal space. Put on some background music such as the instrumental music "On the Day You Were Born."

2. Show the Objects One by One: Pull the first object out of the bag. Ask them, *What is this? How does this object move? Watch while it spins. Can you move like a top? What does the top do when it stops spinning? Can you fall on your side like a top?*

Put the first object away, and pull out the next one. Discuss its properties, and encourage the students to think about the way it moves as they try to move that way themselves.

3. Conclude with a Free Dance: Once you have finished with all of the items in your bag, ask the children if they have a favorite way of moving, and if there is time, let them finish the class with a free dance using ideas from the lesson. Use a lively musical piece, such as "Dancin' Machine." This song gives movement suggestions based on different machines and how they work.

Good-Bye Circle

Ask the students to finish the lesson by thinking of three different ways that they could bow, using three ideas from the lesson today (such as a melting bow like a candle, a spinning bow like a top, and a floating bow like a feather).

Notes

What was successful about this lesson?

Which ideas could have worked better? How could they be improved?

What ideas were generated by the children during the lesson?

How would you enhance or expand this lesson in the future?

Numbers

This lesson uses movement to familiarize children with numbers and counting. The children will learn that counting can be used to determine quantity, as they count how many repetitions of each movement they will do. In addition, they will have the opportunity to form number shapes with their bodies, further familiarizing them with how numbers look in the written form.

MUSIC SUGGESTIONS:

General

- Children's songs about numbers or counting

Specific Selections

- "A Song of One" (*Mother Earth*, Tom Chapin, Gadfly, 2001)
- *Numbers* (Sesame Street, Sony Wonder, 1995)
- The Spanish Numba Rumba (*Sesame Street Fiesta Songs*, Sony Wonder, 1998)
- *Counting Games and Rhythms for the Little Ones* (Ella Jenkins, Smithsonian Folkways, 1967)
- "1, 2, Buckle My Shoe" and "Five Little Ducks" (*Children's Songs, A Collection of Childhood Favorites*, Susie Tallman and Friends, Rock Me Baby Records, 2004)

MATERIALS NEEDED:

- Picture book about counting
- The numbers 0 through 9 written on paper, one to each page or file card
- Drum

Early Learning Standards
8A, 8B, 8C

Opening Activity

Move/Freeze Game about Numbers: Start this lesson with a variation of the move/freeze game. Use a song about numbers or counting as an accompaniment, such as "A Song of One" or "Numba Rumba."

When the music is playing, the children may dance freely. Stop the music at various points, and call out a movement command with a number such as *four jumps*, or *three turns*, or *one fall*, during each pause in the music.

Greeting Circle

Let's count out loud together: *How many children are in our class today?*

Movement Exploration

SEATED WARM-UP

With the children still seated in a circle, have them practice these warm-ups:

1. Up and Down: Ask the children to stand up and go back down to the floor in different counts (Example: *I will start with five. Take all five counts to stand up, and all five to go back down*). Gradually decrease the counts so that the children are popping up and down in one count (remind them to catch themselves with their hands and not fall hard on their bottoms when they go down to the floor quickly).

Any of the warm-ups from past classes can be used in the following exercises, and you can reference the number theme by asking the children how many repetitions of each they would like to do. Encourage them to count along with you during the exercises.

2. Body Parts Isolation: Proceed with a body awareness exercise, and count parts of the body together: *How many ears do we have? How many fingers and toes?* Move each part of the body as it is named, such as wiggling the nose or reaching with the fingers and toes.

3. Flex and Point the Feet: With the legs straight ahead and together, move the feet toward and away from you. *Let's count as we do this exercise. We will count the flex as "one," the point as "two," the flex as "three," the point as "four," and continue up to twelve.*

4. Merry-Go-Round: Seated with knees up to chest, use the arms to twirl the body around. *Let's spin around three times in one direction, rest for a few seconds so we don't get dizzy, and then spin three times in the other direction!*

5. Boat: Seated with soles of the feet together and the knees apart, sway from side to side. *We will count all together up to twenty, counting one number for each sway of our bodies* (count slowly). *Now we will do it again, and you can each choose a number to count up to. When we get to that number in our counting, fall out of your boat!* The children will roll onto their backs on their chosen numbers.

MOTOR SKILLS PRACTICE

1. Continue with large motor skills. This section of class also works well for number exploration. Ask the students how many of each movement they want to do. For example: *How many marches should we do? Let's try fifteen, and we will count together as we march.* Repeat with tiptoe walks, slides, gallops, and runs.

2. To finish the motor skills practice, create a movement phrase using several of the skills. For example, the sequence might be: four marches, seven tiptoe walks, five gallops, one slow turning fall to the floor. Use the drum for accompaniment, and call out the sequence slowly as the children do the phrase. Repeat several times.

SHAPING OUR BODIES INTO NUMBERS

1. Show the Written Numbers: Gather the children together, and read the counting book to the children. Then show them the numbers you have written on cards (first in order, and then randomly), and make sure that they are familiar with all of the numbers you

are using. If they are not, pick out three or four that they are able to recognize.

2. Create a Number Shape: Instruct the children to stand up and find a personal space. Hold up one of the number cards, and ask them to shape their own body into that number. Start out with an easy one, like "1," and then, changing cards, call out another number as they attempt that shape. Go through all of the cards with familiar numbers. Remind the students that they should make the shape with their whole bodies, either standing or while on the floor. Try to discourage the children from using only their fingers to make shapes, as this is a whole-body awareness exercise.

3. Free Dance about Numbers: Play "Five Little Ducks" or another selection about numbers or counting, and let the children move freely to the music. Stop the music periodically, calling out one of the numbers that they have practiced, and ask them to form their bodies into that number shape.

Good-Bye Circle

Gather the children into a circle. Finish the class by counting all the children in the circle out loud together. Then count them backward together.

Notes

What was successful about this lesson?

Which ideas could have worked better? How could they be improved?

*What ideas were generated by the children during
the lesson?*

How would you enhance or expand this lesson in the future?

Percussion Sounds

This lesson is an exploration of percussion, or the sound created by striking one object against another. The children will dance to percussion music, learn about rhythms, make percussion rhythms with their hands, voices, and bodies, and make music with a variety of percussion instruments.

MUSIC SUGGESTIONS:

General
• A variety of percussion selections, and one rousing march selection

Specific Selections
• *The Best of Kodo* (Kodo, Tristar, 1994)
• *Percussion Fantasia* (All Star Percussion Ensemble, Fim [1st Impression], 2003)
• *Sousa Marches* (John Philip Sousa, Decca, 1996)

MATERIALS NEEDED:
• A variety of small percussion instruments, for example, triangles, shakers, rain sticks, tambourines, finger symbols, wood blocks, drums, bells, maracas, spoons, castanets, rhythm sticks. If you do not have these instruments, you can simply use wood blocks and spoons, or any other idea you may have that involves striking one object against another
• Tambourine
• Drum

Early Learning Standards
13B, 15A, 15B

Opening Activity: Tambourine Game

This is a game that will challenge the children to recognize specific rhythms and to associate the rhythms with related movements. It is also an opportunity to practice the movement skills they have been learning and to practice moving to a beat.

1. Introduce the Signals: Explain to the children that when the tambourine makes different sounds, it will signal the children to move in different ways. They will watch and listen for the signals, and then perform the appropriate movement. Here are the signals and the corresponding movements to use for this game:

March	Steady tapping on the head of the tambourine in a medium tempo
Turn	Turning the tambourine in your hands
Moving on the floor	Moving the tambourine along the floor
Gallop	Tapping faster in a gallop rhythm (LOUD-quiet, LOUD-quiet)
Run (and/or shake)	Shaking the tambourine
Hop or jump	Holding the tambourine in both hands in front of you and moving it quickly up and down
Freeze (stop cue)	One sharp, loud hit on the tambourine

Introduce the signals one by one to the children and allow them to practice the movement. As in any warm-up, begin slowly and then build up to the faster movements.

2. Play the Tambourine Game: Have the children begin in a personal space. Tap a rhythm, and continue tapping it while the children perform the corresponding movement. In between each of the movement signals, use the freeze signal to indicate a stop before giving the next signal. Present the different signals randomly throughout the game until the children have mastered all of them. Finish the activity with a freeze signal.

Greeting Circle

1. *Do you know what we were exploring during the tambourine game? Rhythms! I was tapping rhythms on the tambourine, and you were moving to them. Rhythms are patterns made of sounds.*

2. Teach a Poem from Ghana: *Let's listen to some of the rhythms in a children's rhyme from Ghana. This rhyme is called "Banana Sweet":*

> Banana sweet
> Banana sweet
> Sweet banana
> Kwah du ye ye ye
> Kwah du ye.

Repeat it, and ask the children to say it with you several times.

3. Repeat with Children Saying "Banana": *Now I will say the rhyme again, but whenever it is time for the word "banana," I will be silent, and you say the word. You start the poem with the word "banana."*

4. Repeat with Clapping: *Now I will repeat the poem one more time, but instead of saying the word "banana," clap the rhythm of the word using three claps. Remember, you will begin the poem by clapping the rhythm of the word "banana."*

Movement Exploration

MOTOR SKILLS PRACTICE

Continue the process of learning rhythm patterns by setting one or two of the large motor skills to a rhythm. When introducing movement phrases with specific counts, it is helpful to say and clap the rhythm of the exercise with the children first, then show the movement, and then put the two together. It may be challenging for the children at first. However, if you continue this process throughout the year, the children will begin to catch on faster and remember them better.

Incorporate rhythm into the large motor skills practice:

1. March for eight counts straight across the floor, then march for eight counts in a circle, and continue all the way across to the other side of the room.

2. Slide: Clap the rhythm of the slide together: LOUD-quiet, LOUD-quiet, LOUD-quiet, SLIDE-and, SLIDE-and, SLIDE. Ask the children to go across the floor, clapping the rhythm while they are sliding.

3. Jump: *I will recite the poem "Banana Sweet" again. This time, every time I say the word "sweet," you clap. Then, let's clap and jump on the word "sweet."* Repeat the poem several times in a row.

WHAT IS PERCUSSION?

1. Percussion Discussion: Gather the children together again, and have a discussion about the term "percussion." An easy explanation is that "percussion" means "to strike," and percussion instruments are those that make a musical sound as the result of a striking motion.

2. Listen and Dance to Percussion Music: Put on one of your musical selections, such as a band from the Kodo CD, and ask the children to think of as many ways they can of moving to the drum music. Then, if you have a very different percussion selection, such as a piece by the All Star Percussion Ensemble, prompt them to move freely to this.

3. Make Percussion Music with Instruments: *Now that we have explored percussion with our bodies, we are going to make percussion music with instruments!* Briefly show the instruments you have brought, and show how each one is a percussion instrument by demonstrating the different ways each one uses a striking motion. If you do not have percussion instruments, you can make your own using wooden blocks and a spoon.

Distribute one instrument to each child, emphasizing that each child will have the opportunity to play each one. Play a march from the Sousa collection, and let the children dance to the music and try out the instrument. After a couple of minutes, redistribute the instruments. Continue until each child has had a chance to try each one.

How would you enhance or expand this lesson in the future?

Teaching Tip: If the class is large, this can be done in smaller groups, and it is helpful to bring a few categories of instruments (such as several bells, several drums, and several shakers). Then one group can play all the bells at once, and then switch to drums, and then finally shakers, until each group has had the opportunity to try each category of percussion instruments.

Good-Bye Circle

Have the children line up behind you, and then lead them in a parade around the room and out of the dancing area as a lively march plays in the background. Encourage the children to use their imaginations and pretend to play any of the percussion instruments they tried out during the lesson.

Notes

What was successful about this lesson?

Which ideas could have worked better? How could they be improved?

What ideas were generated by the children during the lesson?

The Alphabet

This lesson uses movement to familiarize children with the letters of the alphabet. In addition, the children will learn that letters are tied to sounds as they try to guess what letter different movement words begin with. These skills will be useful as the children begin early reading and writing.

MUSIC SUGGESTIONS:

General
- Any children's songs about letters and the alphabet

Specific Selections
- "The Alphabet Song" (*101 Toddler Favorites*, Various Artists, Music for Little People, 2003)
- *Alphabet Songs* (Jim Post, Reading by Ear, 2005)
- Taj Mahal's "Funky Bluesy ABCs" (*Shake Sugaree*, Taj Mahal, Music for Little People, 1988)
- "The Silly Song" (*Dance in Your Pants*, David Jack, Ta-Dum Productions, 2002)

MATERIALS NEEDED:
- Index cards on which you have written all the letters of the alphabet in capitals
- A picture book about the alphabet, such as *Alphabeasts: A Hide-and-Seek Alphabet Book* (Durga Bernhard, Holiday House, 1993), or *Anamalia* (Graeme Base, Harry N. Abrams, 1993)
- Optional: Alphabet poster
- Drum

Early Learning Standards
7A, 7C, 7D

Opening Activity

Free Dance about the Alphabet: Play "The Alphabet Song" from the *101 Toddler Favorites* CD, or a similar alphabet song. Ask the children if they know any of the letters that are being named in the song. Suggest to the children that they are each holding an imaginary pencil, and ask them to write any letters they know in the air while they dance to the song.

Greeting Circle

Read the alphabet book you have brought, showing them the pictures of the letters as you read. You can also show the poster, if you have one. *Let's recite the alphabet together!*

Movement Exploration

WARM-UP

1. Create Letters While Seated: Have the children be seated in a personal space. Show them the index cards you have brought with the following letters: C, I, J, L, O, P, T, U, V, and Y. As you show the cards one by one, ask the children if they can name the letter. Then ask them to make their bodies into that letter shape while either sitting or lying on the floor. Encourage the children to use their whole body, and not just their fingers and hands to make the letter shapes.

2. Create Letters While Standing: Repeat the above activity, with the children standing, using cards with the letters C, J, L, O, D, T, X.

3. Create Letters with a Partner: Continue this exercise having the children work in pairs to create some of the more complex letters: A, B, E, F, G, M, R, H, N, W, K, S, Q, and Z.

MOTOR SKILLS PRACTICE

Naming the Letters That Begin Movement Words: Tie the theme of the lesson into the motor skills practice by asking, *What letter does the word "march" begin with? Tiptoe? Slide? Gallop? Run?* Lead the children in each skill as it is named, traveling from one side of the room to the other.

FREE DANCE

Play another of the alphabet songs. While the music is playing, challenge the children to try to spell out their names with their bodies, or write in the air again with an imaginary pencil.

Good-Bye Circle

Finish the class by spelling out a group word. Help them spell out "DANCE" or "ALPHABET" or a whole sentence, and then ask them to bow in their letter shape.

Notes

What was successful about this lesson?

What ideas were generated by the children during the lesson?

How would you enhance or expand this lesson in the future?

Which ideas could have worked better? How could they be improved?

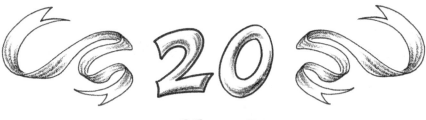

Doodle Bugs

This is a lesson that draws upon many aspects of bugs—types, habitats, physical characteristics—as prompts for movement ideas. The lesson culminates with each child imagining, designing, and dancing about his or her own "Doodle Bug."

MUSIC SUGGESTIONS:

General
- Music or songs about bugs, and one selection of music with a conga rhythm

Specific Selections
- "Flight of the Bumblebee" (*Classical Juke Box, Vol. 1*, Various Composers, Sony, 1991)
- "Doodlebugs" (*Whaddaya Think of That?* Laurie Berkner, Two Tomatoes, 2001)
- "La Cucaracha" (*Children's Songs, A Collection of Childhood Favorites*, Susie Tallman, Rock Me Baby Records, 2004)
- "Conga Line" (*Kids in Action*, Greg & Steve, Greg & Steve Productions, 2000)

MATERIALS NEEDED:
- Paper—any color, 8 x 11 inches or similar size
- Crayons or markers (a variety of colors)

Early Learning Standards
12A, 14A

Opening Activity

Name a Bug! Begin this class by asking the children to move freely to "Flight of the Bumblebee" or a similar selection. Stop the music, and ask a child to name a kind of bug or insect. Start the music again, and ask everyone to move like the bug the child has named. Continue until every child has had the opportunity to name a bug.

Greeting Circle

Did you realize there are so many kinds of bugs? What other ones can you name?

Movement Exploration

SEATED WARM-UP

Bugs provide a wealth of movement images for a fun warm-up:

1. Pill Bug: With the children lying on the floor on their sides, prompt them to curl up and stretch out several times like a pill bug. Repeat, lying on the other side.

2. Upside-Down Bug: Ask the children to roll onto their backs like a bug that is stuck, and exercise their arms and legs by waving them in the air.

3. Inchworm: On hands and knees, stretch arms and pull the body forward like an inchworm.

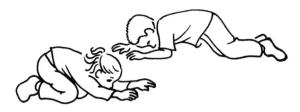

4. Bring the Children to Standing: Ask the children to hop up like a grasshopper, and then jump from blade to blade of grass.

MOTOR SKILLS PRACTICE

1. March: *Let's march like busy ants!*

2. Tiptoe: *Tiptoe like a sneaking bug!*

3. Run: *Let's pretend like we are flying and swooping like a butterfly!*

DOODLE BUGS

1. Create a Bug: Gather the children together. Pass out paper and markers, and ask the children, *If you could imagine a bug, which we will call your "Doodle Bug," what would you like it to be? What color? How big? Would it have wings to fly? Would it have antennae? How many legs would your bug have? Would it be decorated with lots of patterns and colors? What would its face look like?* Give them some time to design their imaginary bugs.

2. Move Like Your Doodle Bug: Put the papers aside, play the song "Doodlebugs," or another lively song, and ask the children to move like their imaginary bugs.

3. Move Like the Other Doodle Bugs: Prompt them to move like some of the other bugs in the classroom. The children's version of "La Cucaracha" on the Susie Tallman CD works well for this activity.

Good-Bye Circle

Ask the children, *Have you ever seen a centipede? It is a bug that has lots and lots of legs, and a very long body. We are going to become a giant centipede!* Line the children up behind you. Walk forward and kick to one side, and then the other, to the beat of Steve & Greg's "Conga Line" or another conga piece.

If there is time, give each child a chance to be the leader. Let the conga line take you out of the dancing area to finish the lesson. Ask the children to wave good-bye as they dance.

Notes

What was successful about this lesson?

Which ideas could have worked better? How could they be improved?

What ideas were generated by the children during the lesson?

How would you enhance or expand this lesson in the future?

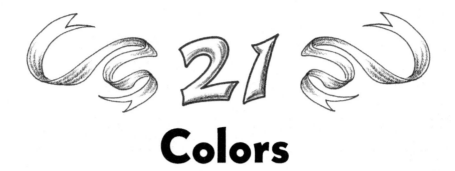

Colors

Exploration of the color spectrum in this lesson spurs a wide range of imaginative movement as the children interpret and react to the different colors. By naming different objects that are all the same color, the children will also learn how to group items that are seemingly different according to one attribute, in this case, color. The children will also learn that different colors can evoke certain emotions.

MUSIC SUGGESTIONS:

General
- Any music that could express ideas and emotions that the children might attribute to colors: classical, blues, drums, New Age, jazz, electronic, etc.
- Any songs about specific colors, all the colors, or rainbows

Specific Selections
- "Many Colores/De Colores" (*Uni Verse of Song: Spanish*, Maria Del Rey, Music for Little People, 1999)
- "Over the Rainbow" (Dan Zanes, *Rocket Ship Beach*, Festival Five Rec., 2000)
- "Colors of the Wind" (*Pocahontas: An Original Walt Disney Records Soundtrack*, Various Artists, Disney, 2001)
- "Blue Danube Waltz" (*Mad About Cartoons*, Various Artists, Deutsche Grammophon, 1993)
- A variety of other selections that have different qualities and tempos, to use while dancing about the various colors

MATERIALS NEEDED:
- Rainbow-colored fabric cut into wide strips, or ribbons of many colors tied together. The prop should be no more than 12 inches long.
- A picture book about color, a color chart, or crayons of many colors
- Drum

Early Learning Standards
9D, 16A

Opening Activity

Free Dance about Colors: Explain that today the children will dance about color. Play "Many Colors/ De Colores," or another selection about colors, and encourage the children to move freely to the music.

Greeting Circle

Gather the children together in a circle and ask, *What is your favorite color?*

Movement Exploration

SEATED WARM-UPS

Begin with seated warm-ups:

1. Merry-Go-Round: Seated with the legs close to the chest, use the arms to spin around several times. *As we turn around one way and then the other, let's imagine colorful animals on a big merry-go-round!*

2. Kitty-Cat: While on hands and knees, arch and curve the back several times. Repeat, incorporating the theme of color: *What color kitty-cat are you?*

3. Bring the Children to Standing: *Okay, colorful kitty-cats, we are going to jump very high! Can you crouch low, and then jump, so that you finish standing up?*

MOTOR SKILLS PRACTICE

Line up on one side of the room and have the children practice these skills as they go across to the other side:

1. March: *March like a toy soldier with a bright red uniform!*

2. Tiptoe Walk: *Walk quietly as a gray mouse on your tiptoes!*

3. Gallop: *Gallop like a shiny black horse!*

4. Slides: *Pretend to hold a big colorful ball between you when you slide across the room with your partner!*

COLOR EXPLORATION

1. Introduce the Colors One by One: Using a book about colors, a color chart, or crayons as a visual aid, introduce one of the colors: *What is this color? How does this color make you feel?* Ask the children to name items of that specific color.

Then play a musical selection, and encourage them to dance freely about that color, varying the music depending on what the children have discussed. Repeat this with a number of different colors.

2. Prop Exploration: Once you have finished exploring many different colors, give the children the opportunity to dance about all the colors using the fabric or scarves.

> **Teaching Tip:** It is best to have all the props the same for each child. Remind the children about the guidelines for working with props: Hold on to the prop while dancing, and do not throw or damage it. If the prop you are using is fabric strips, also remind the children not to tie them or put them around their necks.

Pass out the scarves, and ask the children to find many different ways to move while holding the prop. Prompt the children to remember the large motor skills, like galloping, sliding, and turning as they dance with the props. Encourage variations, such as hop, jump, and fall while holding the prop.

Play one of the musical selections about colors for the prop dance. If there is time, begin with a slower song, such as "Colors of the Wind" or "Over the Rainbow," and then finish with a more upbeat musical selection, such as "Blue Danube Waltz" or other lively classical piece.

Good-Bye Circle

Can you think of a way to bow using your colorful prop?

Notes

What was successful about this lesson?

Which ideas could have worked better? How could they be improved?

What ideas were generated by the children during the lesson?

How would you enhance or expand this lesson in the future?

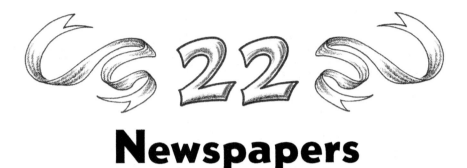

Newspapers

A sheet of newspaper can be a catalyst for a whole gamut of movement activities. The children will explore different shapes by folding and unfolding their newspapers. They will also be thinking about the different ways print can be used by discussing the function of newspapers.

Note: The children can get newsprint on them during the course of this lesson, so a few days before this class, make sure the children have dark play clothes available to wear.

MUSIC SUGGESTIONS:

General
- Bluegrass or other upbeat instrumental pieces

Specific Selection
- "Shuckin' the Corn" and "Orange Blossom Special" (*Bluegrass Breakdown: 14 Instrumentals*, Easydisc, 1997)

MATERIALS NEEDED:
- One double sheet of newspaper for each child, folded to make a single-sized sheet, and one more for demonstration purposes
- Recycling or garbage bag
- Drum

Early Learning Standards
5B, 9A

Opening Activity

1. How Many Shapes from One Page of Newspaper? Hold up one of the folded sheets of newspaper, and ask the children to name the shapes as you make them: First show that it is a rectangle, then fold it to make a square. Rotate the square to show that it is a diamond, and then fold the diamond in half to make a triangle. Finally, scrunch it up to make a circle.

2. Free Dance: Play a selection of upbeat music, and ask the children to move freely to it. Prompt them to use any of the above geometric shapes in their dancing: *Can you move so that your feet follow a rectangle pattern on the floor? A square? A triangle? Can you make circular movements with your body while you move? Can you finish by making a scrunched-up shape in a ball like the newspaper?*

Greeting Circle:

What is a newspaper used for? Do you know any other uses? We are going to explore fun ways to use newspapers today!

Movement Exploration

1. Preparation: Pass out one folded double sheet of newspaper per child. Ask the children to find a personal space in the room and lay the sheet down in their own spaces, keeping it folded.

2. Walk Around: *Can you walk around your sheet of newspaper? Now, try walking around it backward. Now can you walk around it facing forward again, very close to the sheet, but without touching it? Can you do that again, but without looking down?*

3. Make a Bridge: *Try making a bridge over your newspaper with your whole body. Next, try a bridge with only three body parts touching the floor. Now try with five! Can you make a bridge with only two parts touching the floor?*

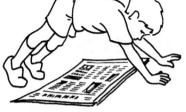

4. Jump Over: *Try jumping over your sheet of newspaper. Can you find two different ways to jump over it?*

5. Roll: *Now try rolling over it. Find three different ways to roll!*

6. Run: *Open up your sheet of newspaper (it will be two full pages now). Run around it without touching it. Run around it three times in a row without stopping!*

7. Scrunch It Up and Make Shapes: *Now we are going to scrunch our newspaper up into a ball. Place it on the floor, let go of it, and watch it open up into a new shape. Can you make the same shape with your body that your newspaper is making?*

Scrunch it up again, curl up next to it, and unfold along with your newspaper into a new shape!

8. Throw It in the Air: *Scrunch it up one more time, into as tight a ball as you can. Throw it up in the air. Can you catch it? Jump as you throw, and try to catch it when you land.*

9. Free Dance with Newspaper: As the children continue this throwing and catching activity, play another track of the bluegrass music, allowing it to evolve into a free dance. At the end of this activity, ask the children to pick up their sheet of newspaper along with any other pieces that have torn off during the lesson.

Good-Bye Circle

Ask the children to bring their pieces of newspaper to you and stand in a circle. Hold a recycling bag, and tell them: *I'm the trash collector! I will come to each of you with my recycling bag. Bow as you throw your paper into my bag!*

Notes

What was successful about this lesson?

Which ideas could have worked better? How could they be improved?

What ideas were generated by the children during the lesson?

How would you enhance or expand this lesson in the future?

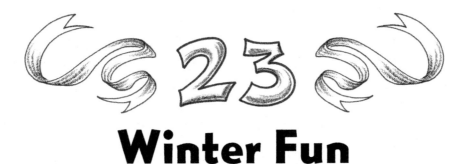

Winter Fun

The winter season inspires variations on many locomotor skills, as well as playful movement games. The children will think about the changing seasons and the characteristics of the winter season. The class ends with an optional story about a girl in South America who sees snow for the first time in her life.

MUSIC SUGGESTIONS:

General
- Melodic instrumental music of moderate tempo
- Several lively selections

Specific Selections
- "As the Snow Falls" (*Winterludes*, The Snowman, Baby Genius, 2003)
- "Cozy Bug Twist" (*Dance in Your Pants*, David Jack, Ta-Dum Productions, 2002)
- "Waltz of the Snowflakes" (*Pytor Illych Tchaikovsky: The Nutcracker—Complete Ballet*, Philips, 1998)
- *Putumayo Presents: Acoustic Brazil* (Various Artists, Putumayo World Music, 2005)

MATERIALS NEEDED:
- Optional: The book *The Town Where It Never Snows* (Paulo Campos, Shinseken Limited, 2001)
- Drum

Early Learning Standards
4C, 12A, 12C

Opening Activity

1. Imagine You're Made of Snow: Stand in a circle with the children and ask them to imagine that they are made of snow. Allow them time to think about being made of big, round snowballs. Then tell them that the sun is coming out, and it's getting warmer. *What happens to snow when the sun shines and it's warm outside?* Encourage the children to slowly melt to the floor.

2. Warm Up Your Body: While sitting, ask the children what happens when it gets really cold: *How does your body react when it is cold? Does it shiver? Let's all shiver! Now let's move each part of our body to try to get warm!* Name each body part as the children warm it up. As each body part is named, the game becomes an isolation warm-up.

3. Snow Wings: *Let's lie down and move our arms up and down to make wing shapes in the snow!*

4. Bring the Children to Standing: *Pretend you are making a small snowball, and then stand up and see how far you can throw your snowball.*

5. Jump: Prompt the children to imagine a large bank of snow that they can jump into or over.

Greeting Circle

What do you see in the winter that is different from other times of the year? What do you like best about winter?

Movement Exploration

MOTOR SKILLS PRACTICE:

1. Walk: Using the image of footprints in the snow, ask the students to imagine that they can see their footprints, and then ask them to retrace their own footprints.

2. Lunge: *Imagine we just had a snowfall, and it is almost over our heads. Let's try to walk through it. It is difficult! We have to take large, heavy steps.*

3. Gallop: *Gallop like a reindeer through a field of snow!*

4. Run: *Let's pretend to run through a blizzard, with lots of wind and blowing snow!*

WINTER EXPLORATION:

1. Footprints in the Snow: Pair the children up in groups of two or three. Elaborating on the idea of footprints in the snow, ask one child from each pairing or group to walk a winding floor pattern, with the other child or children behind him trying to step in his imaginary footprints. Play "Cozy Bug Twist" or another lively selection for this activity. At different points in the song, change the order of the partners so that everyone has an opportunity to lead.

2. Figure 8s on the Ice: This activity is for the children to do individually. Ask the children to imagine they are ice skating. Prompt them to imagine that their skates make visible tracks on the ice, and then suggest geometric shapes that they can make: circles, rounded zigzags, figure 8s. Prompt them to outline the shapes moving forward and then backward. Play a melodic song of moderate tempo, such as "As the Snow Falls," from the *Winterlude* CD, or a similar selection.

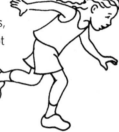

Finally, allow the children to skate freely as you play "Waltz of the Snowflakes" from *The Nutcracker Suite*, or another upbeat classical piece.

3. Read the Story: Gather the children together and read the book *The Town Where It Never Snows*. If you don't have the book, talk to the children about what it is like (if they live in a warm climate), or would be like to never see snow (if they live in a place where there are cold winters). *Can you imagine how happy you would be to see it for the first time?*

4. Free Dance: In the story, it snows in Lucy's town for the first time anyone can remember, and all of the children run out to the park to make snow people. Play a selection from *Putumayo Presents: Acoustic Brazil* while the children dance about wishing for years that they could play in the snow, and finally experiencing snow for the first time.

Good-Bye Circle

Let's each roll a pretend snowball and make a huge snow person using all of our snowballs! How high can we reach to stack all of our snowballs one by one? Now let's sit in a circle around our snow person, and then gently fall backward into the snow. Make snow wings one more time!

Notes

What was successful about this lesson?

Which ideas could have worked better? How could they be improved?

What ideas were generated by the children during the lesson?

How would you enhance or expand this lesson in the future?

24

A Trip around the World

This lesson takes the children on an imaginary vacation. The children will learn about different types of geography and the people and animals that inhabit them. Visit the places described in the lesson plan, or any other places the children are studying or would like to discover.

MUSIC SUGGESTIONS:

General
- Any available ethnic music or songs about traveling
- A lullaby

Specific Selections
- "Places in the World" (*Teaching Peace*, Red Grammer, Red Note, 1986)
- *Putumayo Presents: Africa* (Various Artists, Putumayo World Music, 1999)
- "Me Gusta (I Like It)" (*Sesame Street Fiesta Songs*, Sony Wonder, 1998)
- *Around the World and Back Again* (Tom Chapin, Sony, 1996)
- "Penguin Parade" and "Safe at Home" (*Penguin Parade*, Banana Slug String Band, Warner Bros., 1996)

MATERIALS NEEDED:
- Drum
- Optional: Any books or pictures that show different countries of the world

Early Learning Standards
21B, 21D

Opening Activity

1. Get Ready for the Trip: Ask the children:
Would you like to pretend that we are going on a vacation together? Let's each pack a suitcase! What would you put in your suitcase?

Now let's put our suitcases in our car. It is here in the middle of the room. Have the children pretend to put their suitcases in the car and then make a line behind you in the middle of the room.

2. Imaginary Car Trip: For this activity, you will be taking an imaginary road trip and dropping each child off at his or her own vacation spot. With the children lined up behind you, walk in a line or a loosely structured group and ask each child where she would like to go for her vacation. Make stops every so often to drop off each child at her vacation spot. Let each child leave the group one by one and then come back into it as you continue to drive around the room. Make it fun by waving to the children as you drop them off, and asking them how their vacation was when the group "car" picks them back up. Play "Places in the World" or an upbeat musical selection for this activity.

Greeting Circle:

Did you enjoy our pretend vacation? We are going to visit lots of other places in our class today. Where do you think we will go?

Movement Exploration

MOTOR SKILLS PRACTICE

Practice these large motor skills, traveling from one side of the room to the other:

1. Walk: Instruct the children to follow you in a normal walk across the floor. Then ask them if they can each think of another way of walking. For example, ask if they can use their arms, legs, bodies, heads, etc., in a way that will change the way they usually walk. Prompt them with ideas, such as, *What if you walked without bending your legs? What if you walked by lifting one leg high?*

Variation: Ask each child to think of a different way to walk, and have the class try each child's idea.

2. Repeat with other motor skills. Continue the above idea with any of the motor skills with which the children are familiar: march, tiptoe walk, lunge, slide, gallop, run, jump, or hop.

A TRIP AROUND THE WORLD

The rest of the class will be an imaginary journey to many different lands beginning at the South Pole. Structure this section based on your musical selections, incorporating any additional countries for which you have music along the way. If you have any books or pictures about the countries you will be visiting, read or show them to the children as you travel to each place.

Here is an idea of how to structure a journey:

1. South Pole: Tell the children that you will be beginning at the South Pole. Use the music "Penguin Parade" from the CD of the same name. Ask the children, *Do you know how to march like penguins? Let's pretend to be floating on an ice floe. Look down into the water. What do you see?*

2. Row to the Sahara Desert: Have the children sit on the floor in a line behind you and "row" to another place, such as the Sahara Desert in Africa. Use musical selections from the Putumayo CD *Africa*, or similar music. Prompt them with movement ideas about animals that they might see in the desert. *Let's pretend we are camels in the Sahara!*

3. Fly to Mexico: Gather the children together again and ask them if they would like to visit Mexico. Ask them if they would like to fly in an airplane to get there. For the airplane, simply have the children form a line behind you and move around the classroom. Ask the children to look out of the window and talk about what they see below. Once they arrive in Mexico, play "Me Gusta" ("I Like It"), or other music with a lively Latin beat, for a free dance about Mexico.

4. Continue the Journey: Dance about as many places as time allows, using many different forms of transportation, and incorporating suggestions from the children.

5. Return Home: Finish this section of the lesson with a free dance to "Around the World and Back Again" from the Tom Chapin CD of the same name, or any similar song about traveling.

Good-Bye Circle

Play the song "Safe at Home" from the *Penguin Parade* CD, or a similar lullaby-type song, and ask the children to lie down as if they were back home in their very own beds.

What was successful about this lesson?

Which ideas could have worked better? How could they be improved?

What ideas were generated by the children during the lesson?

How would you enhance or expand this lesson in the future?

Balloons

This lesson uses the characteristics and qualities of balloons to spur movement ideas. The activities in this lesson are designed to reinforce the idea of movement quality as the children practice being "filled with air" and then "popping." The class ends with two lively movement games using the balloons. The children will also continue to practice using props safely and responsibly.

Note: Before teaching this class, make sure that the children are able to understand that balloons should not be placed near the face.

MUSIC SUGGESTIONS:

General
- Several upbeat selections, such as ragtime, classical, and music with a rock and roll beat

Specific Selections
- "Bop 'Til You Drop" (Nylons, *One Size Fits All*, Windham Hill Records, 1990)
- "Palm Leaf Rag" (Coleman, Joplin, *The Complete Rags of Scott Joplin*, Music Masters Jazz, 1995)
- "William Tell Overture" (Various Composers, *Thunderous Classics*, Cincinnati Pops Orchestra, Vox, 2000)

MATERIALS NEEDED:
- A bag of long, wavy balloons, one per child (and a few extras). Blow the balloons up, but not too tight; they last longer if they are not blown up to full capacity
- Drum

Early Learning Standards
10C, 22C

Opening Activity

1. Pretend You Are a Balloon: Begin this lesson with the children standing in their personal spaces. Ask the children to imagine that they are a balloon: *If you were a balloon, what color would you be? What shape? How big?*

2. Floating: *Now I am going to pretend to fill each of you up with air.* Go to each child and pretend to fill him or her up with air. Tell the children, *Once you are filled with air, you can begin to float. What do you see far down below? What do you see up in the sky? Are you floating in and out of the clouds?*

3. Pop! *When I call your name and hit my drum once loudly, that means you will pop and fall to the ground.* Call each child's name one by one, and as you do, the child should fall to the floor in a controlled way. This activity works well with lively music, such as "Palm Leaf Rag."

Greeting Circle

Sit in a circle with the children and discuss the movement quality of balloons: *Is a balloon light or heavy? Before it is blown up, is it floppy? While it is being blown up, is it stretchy? After it is blown up, do you know why it is so light?*

MOTOR SKILLS PRACTICE

Practice large motor skills using balloons as a reference:

1. Walk: *Can you walk heavily, and then as light as a balloon?*

2. Tiptoe Walk: *Can you walk lightly on your tiptoes?*

3. March: *Can you march with your arms in a circle in front of you, like you are holding a round balloon?*

4. Slide: *Can you slide facing your partner, pretending to hold a large round balloon between you?*

5. Gallop and Run: *Can you gallop heavily, and then can you run lightly like a balloon?*

Finish the warm-up with two different balloon activities:

6. Up and Down: Ask the children to lie down in a personal space. Then tell them, *Slowly come to standing as if you are being filled with air like a balloon.* You can make blowing noises to help them imagine it. Once they are all standing, say, *Oops, someone popped you! You have to fall down!*

Repeat this several times. Then vary it, with these ideas: *What if someone blew you up very slowly? Very quickly? Then what if someone let the air out of you very slowly? Very quickly? Now pretend to fill up with air one more time, and pop as fast as you can!*

7. A Great Big Balloon: Have the children stand up and make a circle in the center of the room, as if they were one giant balloon. Prompt them to imagine the air going out of this big balloon, and guide them to close in the circle. Then prompt them to imagine that a giant is blowing up the balloon, and guide the children to open out into a very large circle. Repeat with the different movement ideas from the last exercise (fast, slow, and popping).

BALLOONS

1. Introduce the Balloons: Now gather the children together and pull one of the wavy balloons out of the bag. Explain to the children that balloons are safe to use as long as they never put a balloon close to their mouths. If that happens, discontinue this activity. This is a very important safety issue.

2. Pair Balloon Pass: Distribute one balloon to every two children, and space the groups out around the room. Ask each pair to try to pass the balloon to each other in the air. The song "Bop 'Til You Drop" works well with this activity.

3. Individual Balloons in the Air: For the last activity, distribute a balloon to each child. Ask them, *Can you keep your balloon up in the air? How long can you keep it up before it falls to the floor?* Play the "William Tell Overture" as the accompaniment for this activity. If the class is very large, divide it into smaller groups. Give the children in each group the opportunity to try to keep their balloons in the air, while the rest of the children watch as an audience. Collect all of the balloons at the end of this activity.

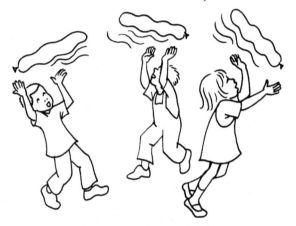

Stand in a circle with the children and say, *Let's pretend we are balloons that have been filled tight with air, and as the air slowly goes out, we will melt to the floor.*

What was successful about this lesson?

Which ideas could have worked better? How could they be improved?

What ideas were generated by the children during the lesson?

How would you enhance or expand this lesson in the future?

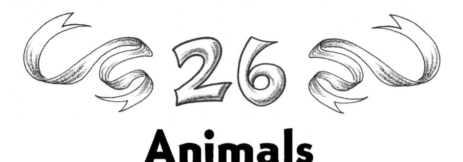

Animals

The animal kingdom provides a wealth of movement ideas, which are explored in this lesson and in Lesson 27. By exploring different animals and the way they move, the children will be expanding their knowledge of the natural world around them. The children will also engage in dramatic play, as the lesson concludes with an action-packed dance story based on a folktale from the Limba of Sierra Leone.

MUSIC SUGGESTIONS:

General

- A song about animals
- African music for background in the dance story

Specific Selections

- Mookie Pookie Choo Choo Choo (*Dance in Your Pants*, David Jack, Ta-Dum Productions, 2002)
- *Putumayo Presents: Africa* (Various Artists, Putumayo World Music, 1999)

MATERIALS NEEDED:

- Optional: The book *Mabela the Clever* (Retold by Margaret Read MacDonald, Albert Whitman & Company, 2000)
- Drum

Early Learning Standards
4C, 10C, 12A

Opening Activity

Free Dance about Animals: Play a musical selection that has references to many kinds of animals, such as "Mookie Pookie Choo Choo Choo." If you do not have a musical selection that mentions animals, you can show pictures of animals from a magazine or book. Prompt the children to think about how each animal moves and suggest that they incorporate these ideas into their own movements.

Greeting Circle

Seated in a circle, ask the children, *Have you ever seen animals in the neighborhood where you live?*

Movement Exploration

SEATED WARM-UP

Begin with a short warm-up using the animal theme:

1. Upside-Down Bug: While lying on the back, move the arms and legs in the air.

2. Cobra: Lying face down, place hands flat on the floor near shoulders, with elbows close to the body. As you press the tops of the feet into the floor, breathe in and lift the chest a couple of inches off the floor. The head stays in line with the spine, and the elbows stay bent and close to the body. Slowly breathe out and lower to the floor. Repeat several times.

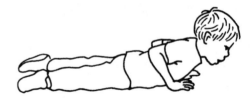

3. Lizard Crawl: Lying face down, bend one leg up and to the side, then use the arm and bent leg on that side to propel the body forward. Repeat on the other side, and continue moving forward by alternating sides.

4. Kitty-Cat: While on hands and knees, arch and curve the back.

5. Downward Facing Dog: This is a position in which the body is supported equally on the hands and feet. Hands are shoulder-width apart, and feet are hip-width apart. The hips are high in the air. The knees can bend as needed.

6. Bring the Children to Standing: From the downward dog position, walk the hands back to the feet, bend the knees, and slowly stand up by uncurling the back.

MOTOR SKILLS PRACTICE

Have the children line up on one side of the room and practice these motor skills to the other side of the room.

1. Prance: The prance is a modified run, in which the body is held very tall. The knees are lifted and stay in front of the body, and the feet land on the toes to the ball to the heel. The knee bend on the landing leg is very small as compared with a normal run. Prances are usually performed at a moderate speed. The image of a horse prancing is helpful in the teaching of this skill. You may want to practice this skill first yourself before introducing it to the children.

2. Jump: *Let's think about how frogs jump! They use their back feet to take off, and as they jump, they move forward, using their front feet to help. Can you crouch low, with your hands on the floor in front of you, and take off into a big jump like a frog? Do it again!* Practice this skill all the way to the other side of the room.

THE TRICKY CAT AND THE CLEVER MOUSE

1. Read the Book or Tell the Story: Gather the children together and read the book *Mabela the Clever*. If you do not have it, you can tell the story yourself, explaining to the children that it is a folktale from Sierra Leone, and it is about learning to be very, very careful:

Once upon a time, there lived a tricky cat, and many foolish mice. But there was one mouse who was not so foolish. Her name was Mabela. Her father told her: *Listen with your ears, look around with your eyes, and pay attention. And if you need to move, move fast!*

The tricky cat came to the mice one day, and said: *You can join our secret cat club. Follow me to my home in the forest, and I will make you members of our club.* The mice lined up, and the cat told them he would march behind them. He also told them they must never look back.

Mabela was in the very front of the line. The mice were marching for a long, long time. But suddenly Mabela remembered what her father had told her: *Listen, look, and pay attention.* She stopped. She listened with her ears, turned around and looked with her eyes, paid attention, and suddenly realized that the line of mice marching behind her was getting smaller. The cat was catching the mice one by one and putting them into his bag! The cat almost caught Mabela, but she remembered her father's other words: *Move fast!*

The cat ran after her, but Mabela was too fast. The cat ended up in a thorn bush, and all the mice got out of the bag and ran away. Mabela saved them all because she remembered to listen, look, pay attention, and move fast!

2. Dance Story: Play a selection from the Putumayo CD *Africa*, or other music from Africa. Ask the children to go to a personal space and to imagine that they are little mice. Begin by reminding them of what Mabela's father told her, adding gestures: *Listen with your ears* (put hands behind the ears with palms out), *look with your eyes* (place hands palms down over the eyes, as if looking into the distance), *pay attention* (stand very still), and *move fast* (run around the room, staying in control). Try repeating the words and gestures several times.

3. Line Up and March: This part of the activity is a variation of a game that was suggested by Margaret Read MacDonald in the introduction to *Mabela the Clever*. Have the children form a line, imagining that they are mice. The teacher will be the cat and will stand at the end of the line. Once the line begins to march, tell the children that they mustn't turn around or look behind them!

As the children begin to march, the teacher says, *Caught you* to the child in front of her, and that child goes to a line that begins to form behind the teacher. This continues until all the mice but the one in the very front are caught. When there is only one mouse left, the teacher signals to all the children to run free. Allow the children a short time to move to the music in a free dance.

Finish the story by stopping the music, and have the children repeat the four gestures from the dance story as you say the following: *Mabela saved all the mice because she listened, looked, paid attention, and moved fast! What a clever mouse, to outsmart the tricky cat!*

Good-Bye Circle

Ask each child to think of an animal, and then bow the way that animal would bow.

Notes

What was successful about this lesson?

Which ideas could have worked better? How could they be improved?

What ideas were generated by the children during the lesson?

How would you enhance or expand this lesson in the future?

More and More Animals

This lesson uses small stuffed animals as props, which stimulate many different movement ideas. As in the last lesson, the children will have the chance to explore how different animals move. In doing so, they will learn to observe differences and similarities between the animals.

MUSIC SUGGESTIONS:

General
- At least one upbeat instrumental selection, and two songs about animals

Specific Selections
- "You Can't Make a Turtle Come Out" (*Grandma's Patchwork Quilt: A Children's Sampler*, American Melody, 2003)
- "Rhinoceros Tap" and "Barnyard Dance" (*Rhinoceros Tap*, Sandra Boynton, Rounder/Pgd, 2004)

MATERIALS NEEDED:
- Bag of small stuffed animals, one per child. Include animals from all categories, such as fish and other underwater animals, sea and land mammals, snakes, lizards, insects, and birds (one per child). If you don't have stuffed animals, you could substitute small plastic animals, but animals that have parts you can move work best.
- Drum

Early Learning Standards
11B, 12A

Opening Activity

Little Turtles: Have the children sit down in their personal spaces. Ask the children to imagine that they are turtles hiding inside their shells. Play "You Can't Make a Turtle Come Out" or an upbeat instrumental selection.

While the music is playing, use the following prompt: *Little turtles, stick out one foot! Uh-oh! You must not want to come out yet, because your foot went back in. Try again! Now try another foot. Poke out your head! Now your tail! Look, you finally came out of your shells! Now you can move all around the room, little turtles.*

Greeting Circle

Bring out your bag of small stuffed animals. Pass the bag around the circle, and allow each child to choose an animal from the bag. Once everyone has an animal, go around the circle and ask each child to tell a little bit about some of the characteristics of their animal. *What is it called? What sound does this animal make? Where does it live?*

Movement Exploration

SEATED WARM-UP

Incorporate the animals in a few short warm-up exercises:

1. Boat: Sit with legs crossed or soles of the feet together and rock from side to side, placing the animal on the floor in the "boat," giving the animal a "ride."

2. Merry-Go-Round: Also while sitting, have the children bring their knees to their chests and spin around on their bottoms several times using their arms to propel them. Then have them spin their animals around the same way.

3. Body Part Isolation: Ask the children to put their animals next to them. Lead the children in a body part warm-up, beginning with the face, and then neck, shoulders, arms, hands, torso, legs, and feet. Then ask the children to help their animals do the same thing, moving the parts of the animals as you say them again.

4. Bring the Children to Standing: Have the children begin in the downward dog position (weight equally on hands and feet, with hips high in the air). Walk the feet forward to the hands, bend the knees, and slowly uncurl the back.

MOTOR SKILLS PRACTICE

For the large motor skills practice, ask the children to line up on one side of the room, carrying their animals while they move across the floor:

1. March: *Can you march, stamping your feet like a great big dinosaur?*

2. Tiptoe Walk: *Can you tiptoe quietly like a mouse?*

3. Prance: *Prance like a proud horse!*

4. Gallop: *Gallop like a zebra!*

5. Run: *Can you run quickly and quietly like a leopard or a cheetah?*

6. Jump: *First, let's all jump up and down while we are holding our animals. Now, standing still, let's throw the animals up in the air and catch them, so they can "jump" too!*

ANIMAL DANCE

1. Dance for the Animals: Line the animals up against a wall of the room, telling the children the animals will be the "audience." Then ask each child to take turns leading the class in the movement of his or her chosen stuffed animal. Play "Rhinoceros Tap" or a similar piece. Continue this activity until every child who wants to has had a chance to lead the class.

2. Dance with the Animals: Now have the children pick up their animals. Suggest to them that they are going to do a good-bye dance with their animals. Prompt them to find as many ways to dance with their animal as they can, using many different movements. Play "Barnyard Dance" for this activity, or repeat "Rhinoceros Tap," or another lively selection.

Good-Bye Circle

Have the children bring their animals into the closing circle. Tell them, *Hold your animal in your hands away from your body, and as you bow, have your animal bow toward you!*

Notes

What was successful about this lesson?

Which ideas could have worked better? How could they be improved?

What ideas were generated by the children during the lesson?

How would you enhance or expand this lesson in the future?

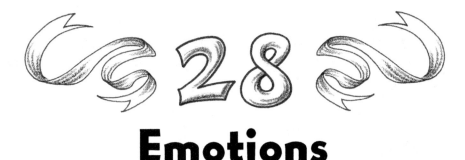

Emotions

This class encourages the children to express feelings and emotions through movement and movement games. The children will learn that different emotions can be expressed through facial expressions, gestures, and movement, all of which are important skills in a child's social and emotional development.

MUSIC SUGGESTIONS:

General
- Different musical selections that could accompany movement about different emotions, such as upbeat, blues, drums, and electronic music

Specific Selections
- "Feelings" (*Getting to Know Myself*, Hap Palmer, 1972)
- "Don't Worry, Be Happy" (*Simple Pleasures*, Bobby McFerrin, Capitol, 1990)
- Blues or sad music, such as "A Soulful Tune" (*Shake Sugaree: Taj Mahal Sings and Plays for Children*, Music for Little People, 1992)
- Music with a driving beat, such as "Home Computer" (*Computer World*, Kraftwerk, Elektra/Wea, 1990)
- Drum music, such as Kodo (*The Best of Kodo*, Tristar, 1994)

MATERIALS NEEDED:
- Pictures of faces with different emotions, such as magazines or books, or the "How Are You Feeling Today?" poster by Jim Borgman (or a copy of it)
- Drum

Early Learning Standards
17A, 15A

Opening Activity

Free Dance about Feelings: Briefly explain to the children that today is a class about feelings. Put on the Hap Palmer song "Feelings" and let the children move freely to the music. If you do not have this song, play an instrumental selection and ask the children to move the way the music makes them feel.

Greeting Circle

Show the children the book or magazine pictures of people with different emotions. Help them to name each one, concentrating mostly on the basic ones that they can readily identify, such as happy, sad, angry, excited, scared, shy, silly.

Movement Exploration

1. Try Out the Feelings on Your Face: With the children seated in a circle, continue to explore the ideas you just discussed. Ask the children to warm up their faces by trying out some of the emotions: *Can you make a happy face? Scared? What about if you feel shy?*

2. Expressing Feelings through Gestures: After trying out emotions through facial expressions, ask the children if they know how to say "I don't know" without using words. They will probably figure out the gesture of moving the shoulders up and down.

Explain to the children how sometimes we express ideas with our bodies and not with words. Ask the children to try to say "yes" and "no" in different ways, using the movements of the body, but without their voices.

3. More Gestures While Standing: Stand up, and now encourage them to put their whole bodies into each of the different emotions. For example, "angry" can be expanded from a simple shake of the head, to crossing arms and making a defiant face, and finally, stamping feet on the floor. "Happy" can begin with a smile and culminate in jumping for joy.

GROSS MOTOR SKILLS

Try an emotion with each large motor skill:

1. Walk: *Walk like you are sad.*

2. March: *March like you are angry.*

3. Tiptoe: *Tiptoe like you are shy.*

4. Gallop: *Gallop like you are happy.*

5. Run: *Run like you are scared.*

6. Slide: *Face your partner while you slide, and make silly faces at each other.*

7. Jump around the room: *Let's make a silly face each time we are in the air!*

DANCE ABOUT DIFFERENT EMOTIONS

1. Happy Dance: The rest of the lesson will be an exploration of four emotions more fully. Begin with "happy," and play "Don't Worry, Be Happy," or a similar selection. Ask the children to think of things that make them happy, and tell them that this is the time to dance about them.

2. Sad Dance: Do the same for "sad," with the Shake Sugaree, or blues, selection.

3. Angry Dance: Follow with "angry," with the Kodo or other drum music.

4. Silly Dance: Finish with "silly," using the Kraftwerk or other music with an electronic, driving beat.

Good-Bye Circle

Bring the children together and take a moment to ask the children how they feel now, and if it is different from the way they felt at the beginning of the class. Ask them to bow in a happy, then sad, then silly way.

Notes

What was successful about this lesson?

Which ideas could have worked better? How could they be improved?

What ideas were generated by the children during the lesson?

How would you enhance or expand this lesson in the future?

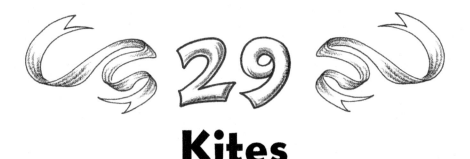

Kites

The children will move like kites dancing in the wind in the spring sky. In doing so, the children will learn about kites, wind and air, and about the ways wind can affect different objects.

MUSIC SUGGESTIONS:

General
- Songs about spring, the wind, or kites

Specific Selections
- "Fly Away" (*All the Colors*, Jim Salestrom, Moulin d'Or, 1997)
- "Let's Go Fly a Kite" (*Mary Poppins*, Disney, 2001)
- "I Am the Wind" (*Toddler's Next Steps: Earth, Moon, & Stars*, Various Artists, St. Clair Records, 2002)

MATERIALS NEEDED:
- Colorful cloth or crepe paper streamers (for kite tails, about 12 inches long)
- Books about kites and wind, such as *Wind* (Ron Bacon, Scholastic, Inc., 1984)
- Poems about kites and wind, such as "For Keeps" by Jean Conder Soule, and "March Wind" by Lee Bennett Hopkins
- Pictures of kites, if you don't have a picture book
- Drum

Early Learning Standards
4C, 12A, 12B

Opening Activity

Free Dance about Spring: Begin this lesson by asking the children what they like about this time of year. Play "Fly Away" or other lively music and let them improvise to their ideas in a free dance.

Greeting Circle

Have you noticed any signs that spring is coming?

Movement Exploration

SEATED WARM-UP

Incorporate ideas that the children have brought up during the Greeting Circle into warm-up exercises for today. Here are some suggestions:

1. Upside-Down Bug: Lie on the back and move the arms and legs back and forth in the air. *Let's be bugs stuck on our backs! Have you seen any bugs yet this spring?*

2. Upper-Body Circling: Seated with legs crossed, move the upper body to the side, forward, to the other side, and back to the upright position. Repeat to the other side. Try it again, this time holding the arms in a round shape overhead, like the sun.

3. Bring the Children to Standing: *Let's stand up very slowly, like a flower growing. Now let's go back down, and come up to standing quickly, like a frog jumping!*

MOTOR SKILLS PRACTICE

Below are some ideas of images to use for the large motor skills. Ask the children for their own suggestions as well.

1. Walk: *We can walk outside without our coats on! Feel the warm spring air as you walk.*

2. March: *Like busy ants!*

3. Slide: *Facing a partner, make a big sun shape with your arms. Try to hold the circle as you slide!*

4. Gallop: *Gallop like a deer through a field of wildflowers!*

5. Run: *Like the wind! Feel the strong wind on your face and arms.*

KITES

Have the children sit in a circle with you as you talk about kites:

1. Read about the Wind: Read a book or poem about the wind, or simply talk about what it is like to be outside in the wind, just as they imagined when they were running.

2. Talk about Kites: Tell the children that you want to discuss something special that likes to dance in the wind. Ask the children, *Can you name some things that like to dance in the sky?* (Examples you can give them are flags, birds, butterflies, leaves, trees). *Is there anything else you can think of?* If they haven't guessed "kites" yet, give them a clue, such as that it can be made of bright colors, or that it has a tail.

3. Read about Kites: Once they have guessed, read your kite poems or book, or show them pictures.

4. Movement Quality of Kites: Continue to spur their imaginations with questions: *Does a kite fly up high? Does it move up and down, side to side, all around? Does it move fast or slowly? Are its movements smooth or jerky? Light or heavy? Big or little? Has anyone ever held on to a kite while it is up in the air, and felt its tug and pull as it dances in the wind?*

5. Imagine You Are a Kite: With the children still seated in a circle, ask them, *Would you like to be a kite for a little while today? What color kite would you like to be? What shape kite? How big? What would your tail look like?*

6. Kite Dance in Two Groups: The first kite dance will be in two groups, the "kites" and the "holders." Divide the class into two groups. Line the holders up near the edge of the dancing space, and tell them to hold tight to imaginary strings. The kite group will line up in front of the holders. When the music begins, the kite group will run forward and pretend to take off into the air, and then dance as if they were kites flying in the sky. Remind them of the movement ideas you discussed: smooth, jerky, light, heavy, fast, slow, etc. A good accompaniment for this activity is "Let's Go Fly a Kite." Once the song is over, switch groups and repeat this activity so that all the children have a chance to be both kites and holders.

7. Group Kite Dance: The second kite dance is for everyone all together. Pass out the colorful cloth or crepe paper streamers you have brought, and prompt the children to pretend that these are their tails as they dance in the sky. Play the song "I Am the Wind," or similar music, reminding them to stay in their bubbles of personal space as they move about the room, and to use the props responsibly.

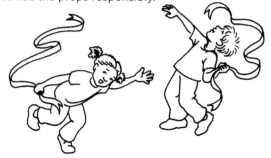

Important Note: When using scarves or strips of cloth, explain two safety guidelines to the children: 1) Don't tie any knots in scarves or tie them to your body, and 2) don't place a scarf around the neck.

Good-Bye Circle

Bow like a kite swirling in the wind!

Notes

What was successful about this lesson?

Which ideas could have worked better? How could they be improved?

What ideas were generated by the children during the lesson?

How would you enhance or expand this lesson in the future?

30
"The Ugly Duckling"

The classic "Ugly Duckling" tale inspires a dance story. The children will have the chance to engage in dramatic play as they move like ducklings, and, in the process, they will be learning about the natural world and the cycle of life.

MUSIC SUGGESTIONS:

General
- A song about birds or flying, if available
- A quiet, rhythmic piece
- A lively classical piece

Specific Selections
- "Like a Bird in the Sky" (Rachel Sumner, *I've Got Imagination*, Rachel's Record, 1997)
- *Winter into Spring* (George Winston, Windham Hill Records, 2002)
- "Swan Lake (Dance of the Swans)" (*25 Classical Favorites*, Various Composers, Vox, 1996)

MATERIALS NEEDED:
- A book or story about "The Ugly Duckling" (if you do not have a picture book, bring a picture of a baby duck, a baby swan, and an adult swan)
- Drum

Early Learning Standards
4C, 12A, 16A

Opening Activity

Have the children stand in their personal spaces. Begin the lesson by asking the children what it would be like to be a baby bird learning to fly. Prompt them with ideas: *First, the bird would waddle and stumble, and then it would spread its wings and try to fly. It flaps its wings hard, but nothing happens! It keeps trying, and then it can*

finally fly up in the air! Play "Like a Bird in the Sky," and let the children dance about this idea.

Greeting Circle

What did it feel like to move as if you were flying?

Movement Exploration

SEATED WARM-UP

With the children seated in a circle, repeat the following warm-up activities from the previous lesson:

1. Upside-Down Bug: Lie on the floor with arms and legs in the air. *Let's be bugs stuck on our backs! Have you seen any bugs yet this spring?*

2. Upper-Body Circling: Seated with legs crossed, move the upper body to the side, forward, to the other side, and back to the upright position. Repeat to the other side. Try it again, this time holding the arms in a round shape overhead, like the sun.

3. Bring the Children to Standing: *Let's stand up very slowly, like a flower growing. Now let's go back down, and come up to standing quickly, like a frog jumping!*

MOTOR SKILLS PRACTICE

Have the children continue practicing these large motor skills from the previous lesson, traveling together from one side of the room to the other:

1. Walk: *We can walk outside without our coats on! Feel the warm spring air as you walk.*

2. March: *Like busy ants!*

3. Slide: *Make a big sun shape with your partner and try to hold the circle as you slide!*

4. Gallop: *Gallop like a deer through a field of wild-flowers!*

5. Run: *Like the wind! Feel the strong wind on your face and arms!*

THE UGLY DUCKLING:

1. Tell the Story of "The Ugly Duckling":
Gather the children together and read "The Ugly Duckling," or tell the story in your own words and use pictures you have brought.

2. Dance Story: Ask each child to find a personal space in the room. Play a selection from *Winter Into Spring*, or a similar piece, softly for background music. Narrate as the dance begins and encourage the children to move to the narration:

> You are a baby bird inside of an egg. Very carefully try pecking on the inside of your shell with your beak. Is it time to come out? Try to stick out one of your webbed feet. You have to work hard! Push the other one through. Can you push your tiny wing out? The other wing? How about your beak? Now pop all the way out. Shake out your feathers!
>
> Try out your beak—can you open it wide? Open and close your eyes. Try flapping your little wings. Move your legs and feet. Look at you, you are a baby duckling! Welcome to the world.
>
> Can you waddle around? Look how clumsy you are because you are so new. But all of the other ducks say that you look different from them, and they want you to go away!
>
> Run away and hide in the tall grass. You are very lonely!
>
> Now you go for a swim in the cold pond. Uh-oh! The lake is frozen. You are stuck! How will you get out? When you get unstuck, run back to your hiding place in the grass.
>
> When spring comes, you feel stronger. You are ready to try to fly. Spread your wings, run, and take off into the sky. You are flying for the first time! What does it feel like? How high can you go? What do you see up there in the sky?
>
> Come in for a smooth landing onto a pond. While you are swimming around, you suddenly notice some majestic white swans. Now look into the water, where you can see your own reflection. What

do you see? Swim over to the other swans! Now you know that you have found your home. Dance with the other swans! For this last dance, play "Dance of the Swans" or a light, classical piece.

Good-Bye Circle

Take a bow like a shy duckling, and then like a proud swan!

Notes

What was successful about this lesson?

Which ideas could have worked better? How could they be improved?

What ideas were generated by the children during the lesson?

How would you enhance or expand this lesson in the future?

In the Toy Shop

This lesson is an imaginary visit to a toy shop. The different toys inspire various movement qualities, and the class culminates in a dance story. Dance stories are a great way to encourage the children's imagination.

MUSIC SUGGESTIONS:

General
- Music that evokes the feeling of play, toys, and toy instruments

Specific Selections
- "Variations (Twinkle, Twinkle)" (*Baby Einstein: Lullaby Classics*, Buena Vista, 2004)
- "Rag Doll Rag" (*Dance in Your Pants*, David Jack, Ta-Dum Productions, 2002)
- "March of the Toys," "Parade of the Wooden Soldiers," "The Toy Trumpet" (Various Composers, *Classics for Kids*, RCA, 1993)

MATERIALS NEEDED:
- Drum
- Any wind-up toys or toys with moveable parts

Early Learning Standards
16A

Opening Activity

Begin this class by asking the children to name some different kinds of dolls, such as rag dolls, robot dolls, baby dolls, wooden soldier dolls, etc.

Now play "Variations" by Mozart, and prompt them to move as a different doll to each variation. (These are variations of the melody of "Twinkle Twinkle Little Star.") If this music is unavailable, use another playful selection, and call out different dolls throughout the song: *Can you march like you are a robot doll? Now pretend you are a rag doll!*

Greeting Circle

Today we are going to dance about toys. Can you think of a toy that has the same starting sound as your name? (For example, Maria/marbles, William/wagon, Yolanda/yo-yo).

Now let's look at some toys I have brought, and we will watch how they move. Bring out the wind-up or moveable toys and show the children how each one moves. *Later in the class, we will imagine toys like these and dance about them.*

Movement Exploration

SEATED WARM-UP

Use the following images of toys as you progress through the warm-up, seated with the children in a circle:

1. Merry-Go-Round: Seated with the knees to the chest, spin one way, and then the other.

2. Bring the Children to Standing: To go from sitting to standing, use the idea of winding up a jack-in-the-box, and popping up, repeating several times.

MOTOR SKILLS PRACTICE

Practice these skills, traveling together from one end of the room to the other:

1. Walk: *Walk like a wind-up doll!*

2. March: *March straight-legged like a robot.*

3. Turn: *Can you spin like a top across the floor?* Make sure the children practice moving in a controlled way for this exercise.

4. Slide: *Slide facing your partner, pretending to hold a giant ball between you.*

5. Run: *Run like a floppy rag doll.*

6. Jump: *Jump in place like a yo-yo, and then jump all around the room like a bouncing ball.*

DANCE STORY: A VISIT TO THE TOY SHOP

1. Prepare for the Dance Story: Gather the children together, and ask them to imagine what it would be like to visit a magical toy shop. Tell them that they are going to pretend to visit one today. Instruct them to stand behind you, starting on one side of the room.

2. Narrate the Story: *Let's take a walk down the street. Look! There is a toy shop! Let's look inside. It looks like the toymaker is asleep. Let's go inside very quietly and explore. Look at all of these toys!* Ask the children what kind of toys would be in the shop.

Let's see what happens when I touch one of the toys. Remind the children of the toys from the Greeting Circle to prompt their imaginations. *Oh look, it is moving on its own! This must be a very special kind of toy shop. Let's go around the shop, see how many toys there are, and touch each of them until they are all moving!*

At this point in the story, put on some music, such as "The Toy Trumpet," and ask the children to dance about the toys coming to life. They can pretend to be a child in the toy shop and dance about playing with one of the toys you have shown; you can also prompt them to move like one or many different toys.

After they have danced to "The Toy Trumpet," play "Parade of the Wooden Soldiers" or a similar song and prompt them to move like wooden soldiers. Then have them dance like rag dolls to "Rag Doll Rag" or a similar tune.

After the children have moved to several musical pieces, continue the story: *Uh-oh! Everybody freeze! The toymaker is waking up! He didn't realize we were in his shop and that all of his toys were moving and playing with us. Quick! Let's run as fast as we can!* Run back to the place where you started the story to conclude the activity.

Variation: If there is time, play "March of the Toys" or a similar song, and prompt the children to dance about any of the toys from today's lesson.

Good-Bye Circle

We are back from our trip to the toy shop. What was your favorite toy that we danced about today? Can you bow like that toy?

Notes

What was successful about this lesson?

Which ideas could have worked better? How could they be improved?

What ideas were generated by the children during the lesson?

How would you enhance or expand this lesson in the future?

32

Caterpillars and Butterflies

The cycle of metamorphosis from caterpillar to butterfly inspires many imaginative movement ideas. Children will learn about metamorphosis and the natural world as they engage in a dramatic play activity.

MUSIC SUGGESTIONS:

General
- Two upbeat classical pieces, and a quiet background selection

Specific Selections
- "Norwegian Dance" (*Grieg: Greatest Hits*, Edvard Grieg, Sony, 1994)
- "When Bullfrogs Croak" (*When Bullfrogs Croak*, Zak Morgan, Zak Records, 2003)
- "On the Day You Were Born" (instrumental) (*On the Day You Were Born*, Debra Frasier, composed by Matthew Smith, Harcourt Children's Books, 2005) (hardcover and musical CD edition)
- "Gallop" (*Classics for Kids*, Various Artists, RCA, 1993)

MATERIALS NEEDED:
- Drawing paper
- Crayons or markers
- A book or pictures that show the cycle of a caterpillar turning into a butterfly, such as *The Life Cycle of a Butterfly* (Angela Royston, Heinemann Library, 1998)
- Drum

Early Learning Standards
12A, 16A

Opening Activity

Begin this lesson with an imaginary walk outside. Walk around the classroom, pretending that you are all outside admiring the beautiful spring day. Jump over streams, climb hills, pick flowers, feel the wind on your face, wade in a pond. "Norwegian Dance" works very well as an accompaniment for this activity, because it varies from slow to fast throughout the piece. A fun song accompaniment is "When Bullfrogs Croak."

Variation: If you have an outside play area, walk around it instead, noticing flowers, grass, and other natural phenomena.

Greeting Circle

What is your favorite thing to do when you play outside?

Movement Exploration

MOTOR SKILLS PRACTICE

Continue the ideas from the "walk" outside for the warm-up, and then teach a movement sequence by introducing the skills one by one:

1. **Walk** a winding path.

2. **Hop** on stepping stones.

3. **Gallop** across a meadow.

4. **Run and jump** over a stream.

5. **Fall and roll** down a hill.

6. **Dance phrase or sequence:** Once the children have tried each of the above skills, ask them to perform the movements in a sequence: walk, hop, gallop, run, jump, fall, roll. Repeat several times.

Variation: Ask the children to add a freeze shape to the end of the phrase. For example, at the end of the roll, freeze in a final position on the floor to signal the end of the movement sequence.

CATERPILLAR TO BUTTERFLY

1. Prepare for the Dance Story: Gather the children together and read the book or show the pictures you have brought, which illustrate the cycle of a caterpillar turning into a butterfly.

2. Draw a Caterpillar: Next, pass out the drawing paper and crayons or markers. Ask the children to draw a caterpillar. Prompt them: *If you were a caterpillar, what kind would you be? What color? How big? Where would you live?*

3. Dance Story: After they have completed their drawings, put the papers aside, and explain to them that now they are going to pretend to be a caterpillar. Have the children begin in a personal space, and play a long musical selection for background, such as the instrumental music "On the Day You Were Born," and begin:

First, you will start out as a little tiny caterpillar. You are going to have to eat lots of leaves to get really big. Look all around for leaves that caterpillars like to eat.

Once you are very full, find a good stem. Prompt the children to imagine that they are hanging from a stem. *Now you will have to spin your cocoon, because you are ready for your special change into a butterfly. Spin, spin, spin!*

You are completely inside of your cocoon now. We have to wait while you slowly turn into a butterfly. While we are waiting, think about what shape and color you want to be when you come out of your cocoon.

Okay, poke your legs, your head, your wings, out of your cocoon. You are free! But wait, your wings are wet. They have to dry before you can fly. Move into the sun, to help warm and dry your wings. Feel the warm sun on your new wings. Now move your wings very, very slowly. Flap them slowly and gently, and then gradually begin to flap them with more and more energy.

Suddenly, you realize you can fly! Fly all around the room, beautiful butterflies! Change the music to a livelier piece, such as "Gallop," for this last dance.

4. Draw a Butterfly: At the end of the class, gather the children back together and pass their caterpillar pictures back to them. Now ask them to draw the butterfly that they became. Then suggest they take their pictures home, to remind them about the dance story of a caterpillar turning into a butterfly.

Good-Bye Circle

How would you bow if you were a caterpillar? What about a great big caterpillar that has eaten lots of leaves?

Notes

What was successful about this lesson?

Which ideas could have worked better? How could they be improved?

What ideas were generated by the children during the lesson?

How would you enhance or expand this lesson in the future?

More Butterflies

This is a further exploration of butterflies and how they move. The lesson includes a variety of media, movement, music, and two different types of props to enhance the imaginative play. The children will be learning about the natural world as they continue to explore their own bodies in motion.

MUSIC SUGGESTIONS:

General
- Two lively classical pieces, or other up-tempo instrumental music

Specific Selections
- "Flight of the Bumblebee" and "Pizzicato Polka" (*Classical Juke Box, Vol. 1*, Various Composers, Sony, 1991)
- *Respighi: Ancient Aires and Dances* (Ottorino Respighi, EMI Classics, 1998)

MATERIALS NEEDED
- Clothespins (three for each child)
- Pipe cleaners (one for each child)
- Colorful tissue paper cut in ovals about 5 or 6 inches long (two or three per child)
- Colorful scarves or fabric (each about 12 inches square) to be used for "wings" (two fabric squares per child)
- Drum

Early Learning Standards
12A, 16A

Opening Activity

MOTOR SKILLS PRACTICE

These motor skills provide a basis for this opening activity to get the children moving. Repeat the large motor skills practice from last week, with the children traveling together from one end of the room to the other:

1. **Walk** a winding path.

2. **Hop** on stepping stones.

3. **Fall and roll** down a hill.

4. **Gallop** across a meadow.

5. **Run and jump** over a stream.

6. **Try the Movement Phrase.** Combine all of the above skills in a series: Walk, hop, gallop, run, jump, fall, roll. Call out the movements as cues.

Ask each child to think of a way to come to standing after the roll, and that will be each child's new ending of the movement phrase. Now that they have a specific way to stand up, the phrase can be repeated.

7. **Repeat the Phrase:** Ask the children to do the phrase, and repeat it three times in a row, moving around the room. Once they are comfortable with this, play "Pizzicato Polka" or another light classical piece and let the children try the repeated movement phrase with music. As has been stated in similar activities, it is not imperative that the children remember the phrase exactly. It is more important that they try the different movements and are engaged in practicing the motor skills. Continue to call out movement cues, if necessary. Finish the activity with a "freeze" after everyone has come to standing at the end of the last repeat of the phrase.

Greeting Circle

Have you ever seen a butterfly? What color was it?

Movement Exploration

1. Make Clothespin Butterflies: Gather the students together to make small butterflies to use as props. Pass out one clothespin, one pipe cleaner, and two or three tissue-paper ovals per child. The butterfly is easily put together, but the children will need help. Layer the tissue paper together, open the clothespin, and slide the papers in, scrunching the tissue papers in the center where they fit into the clothespin. Fluff them out to make wings once they are secured. Then put the center of the pipe cleaner into the end of the clothespin (by opening it again), and curl the ends up to look like antennae. *Now each child has a butterfly!*

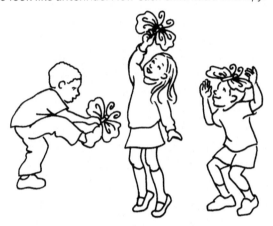

2. Dance with the Butterfly Prop: Suggest a dance that they can do with their butterflies. First ask the children how many ways they can make the butterfly take off and land on different parts of their own body. (For example, *Can your butterfly start on your shoulder, fly through the air, and land on your nose? Can you put your foot in the air and have the butterfly land on it?*)

3. Dance Story: Then prompt the children to dance a story with the butterflies: The children begin seated, with the butterfly resting on a knee. With music in the background, such as a selection from Respighi's *Ancient Aires and Dances*, ask the children to imagine the butterfly taking off into the air, flying slowly, and then landing on a flower. Have it take off again and fly faster, this time landing on a tree. Prompt them to imagine other places the butterfly might fly. At the end of the music, encourage them to think of a final position for themselves and their butterfly. When they are finished with this dance, ask them to find a place at the edge of the dancing area to place their butterfly.

4. Dance with Butterfly Wings: Use a clothespin to attach a "wing" (a scarf or comparable piece of fabric) to each shoulder of all the children. With "Flight of the Bumblebee" or similar lively music as accompaniment, the children can bring the ideas of the last two classes together. Remind them about the caterpillar-to-butterfly cycle from last week, and have them use their "wings" for a final butterfly dance.

Good-Bye Circle

Bow using your big butterfly wings!

Notes

What was successful about this lesson?

Which ideas could have worked better? How could they be improved?

What ideas were generated by the children during the lesson?

How would you enhance or expand this lesson in the future?

The Enchanted Scarves

The simple prop of a scarf can become many things, with the help of a little imagination!

This lesson encourages a great deal of creativity as the children pretend that their scarves are enchanted and can turn into something else. In addition, the opening activity, a mirror game, teaches the children about directionality and movement.

MUSIC SUGGESTIONS:

General
- Three upbeat instrumental selections

Specific Selections
- "I Really Love to Dance" (Laurie Berkner, *Buzz Buzz*, Two Tomatoes, 2001)
- "Peer Gynt—Anitra's Dance" and the "Blue Danube Waltz" (*Mad about Cartoons*, Various Artists, Deutsche Grammophon, 1993)

MATERIALS NEEDED:
- A bag of scarves (as used in Lesson 33), one scarf per child. Sheer, flowing fabric is best, but any soft fabric the size of a scarf (12 inches square) can be used
- Drum

Early Learning Standards
9E, 16A

Opening Activity: The Mirror Game

1. Mirror Game Preparation: Begin this class with a mirror game. This game serves as a warm-up. Place the students in a line (or staggered lines) facing you, making sure there is plenty of space between each child.

2. Mirror Game Explanation: Tell the children that they are going to pretend to look into a very special mirror. The image they will see is you, and they should try to follow your movement as if they were looking into the mirror. Explain it to them by demonstrating, for example, by pointing your right hand to the side, and help them to figure out that they should point their left hands to the side. Lift your left leg, and they should lift their right legs. Walk backward slowly, and help them to understand that they should slowly back away from you, making sure they understand the mirror concept.

3. Play the Mirror Game: Now the children are ready for the mirror game. Begin slowly, standing in one spot facing the children, and move different body parts in many different ways. Speed up your movements, slow them down, stop and start, go down to the floor, jump in the air, etc. If the children are catching on well, you can do more difficult movements, such as turning, moving sideways, and moving away from and toward them. A good accompaniment for this activity is "I Really Love to Dance," because it has changes in tempo, as well as suggestions for different movements. An upbeat instrumental selection works well too.

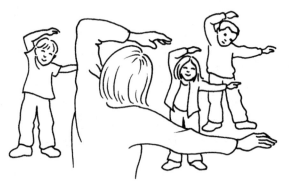

Greeting Circle

Gather the students into a circle, seated on the floor. Tell them that you have a special scarf to show them and that each child can make it into something different. Pull out one of the scarves you have brought. Pass it to the first child, and ask him or her to pretend that it is something other than a scarf (some ideas you can suggest, if they need them, are an apron, a blanket, a tablecloth for a picnic, a cape, a tail, a lasso, a veil, a flying carpet). Make sure that each child in the circle has the opportunity to think of a new idea as well as demonstrate it with the scarf. The children will get many ideas from each other, which they can use in the next activity.

Important Note: When using scarves, explain the two safety guidelines for the children: 1) Don't tie any knots in scarves or tie them to your body and 2) don't place a scarf around the neck.

Movement Exploration

Free Dance with Scarves: Give each child a scarf. The previous activity should have spurred their imaginations with lots of creative ideas for using the scarves. Play "Anitra's Dance," "Blue Danube Waltz," or another lively piece, and prompt the children to think of many ways to use and dance with their scarves. Repeat the safety guidelines above before the free dance begins.

Variation: Try to do this free dance in two groups, one group being an audience while the other group dances. The children will observe each other's ideas and will want to try them out.

Good-Bye Circle

Collect the scarves by having each person bow as he or she places a scarf in your bag.

Notes

What was successful about this lesson?

Which ideas could have worked better? How could they be improved?

What ideas were generated by the children during the lesson?

How would you enhance or expand this lesson in the future?

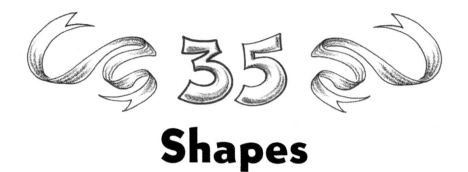

Shapes

This lesson uses movement activities and games to increase the children's recognition and awareness of shape. The children will learn that shapes can come in many forms and that even their bodies can make shapes!

MUSIC SUGGESTIONS:

General:

• Long tracks of upbeat music, such as bluegrass or ethnic

Specific Selections:

• "Foggy Mountain Special" or other selections (*Foggy Mountain Jamboree*, Flatt & Scruggs, County Records, 1993)

• "Sous le Soleil" or other selections (*Presents: World Groove*, Various Artists, Putumayo World Music, 2004)

MATERIALS NEEDED:

• Pipe cleaners, one per child

• Drum

Early Learning Standards
9A, 9C, 9E

Opening Activity

MOVE/FREEZE GAME I

In order to introduce the idea of shape, begin with a move/freeze game. Play "Foggy Mountain Special," or another upbeat musical selection, and give the children a suggestion as to what movement they should start with, such as *gallop*. Then stop the music, and quickly give a shape suggestion. For example, *Freeze by making your body into a wide shape, like a whale. When the music starts again, move only by turning—on the*

floor, in the air, any way you can turn! Call out a different locomotor movement combined with a different shape suggestion each time. To help the children understand the idea of freezing in a very specific shape, use the image of a photograph that catches them in mid-movement. Suggestions for the activity:

Movement Ideas: Walk, turn, move along the floor, hop, jump, march, gallop, slide, tiptoe.

Freeze Shape Ideas: High like a very tall person, low like a snake, curvy like curly hair, twisty like a pretzel, wide like a whale, small like a bug, straight like uncooked spaghetti, crooked like an old tree, one-legged shape like a flamingo.

Finish the game with a final shape, and ask the children to try to hold those shapes as they move to the center of the room. Then ask them to watch how that shape changes as they lower to the floor for the Greeting Circle.

Greeting Circle

Show the children a pipe cleaner. Make a few simple shapes with it, and then pass out a pipe cleaner for each child. Explain in a simple way the connection between the changing shape of the pipe cleaner and the constant changing shapes of our bodies as we move throughout our day. Allow the children a few minutes to manipulate the pipe cleaner, and then collect them. *Today we will be making our bodies into many different shapes, just like the pipe cleaner!*

Movement Exploration

SEATED WARM-UP

This warm-up is structured using basic geometric shapes, with which many of the children will already be familiar, such as circle, triangle, diamond, and star. Have the children sit in a circle with plenty of space between one another.

1. Upper-Body Circle: Sit with legs crossed or in the boat position. Ask the children, *Can you make a circle with your arms to the front? Take the circle shape above the head, and then to the side with your upper body, slowly forward, and then to the other side, and come back up to sitting straight with the circle overhead. Now bring the arm circle in front of you, again, and show how you can make the circle big as you open your arms. Now make it smaller. If you make it small enough, it eventually becomes a hug!*

2. Boat: Sit with the soles of the feet together and the knees apart. *Do you see that when we are in the boat position, our legs make a diamond? Let's imagine that we are taking something in our boat today. What would you like to take? Let's rock back and forth, and see if you can keep a nice diamond shape while we rock.*

3. Straddle Position: From the boat, have everyone open their legs into the straddle position, which is like an open-ended triangle shape. Have the children bring the legs together and apart several times in this position, making a straight line with their legs, and then back to an open-ended triangle.

4. Star: Ask the children to scoot closer together so that everyone's toes are touching, and point out that the shape they all make together is like a many-pointed star. Instruct them to bend their bodies side to side and reach for their toes, and then repeat, reaching for their neighbors' toes.

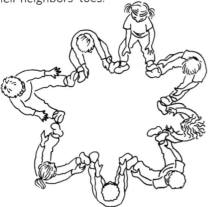

5. Bring the children to standing by asking them to make the circle of children taller.

CHANGING CIRCLE GAME

With the children standing in a circle, ask them, *How could we make the circle bigger?* (They will back away, and because they are moving backward, caution them to look over their shoulders to see where they are going.) Once the circle is as big as the room will allow, ask them, *How could we make our big circle higher?* (They will go up on their toes.) *Lower?* (They should go down to the floor.) *How would you make the circle high, but very small?* (They will go back up onto their toes, and come in very close together.) If this game is working well, you can continue it with different combinations of big, small, high, medium, and low.

MOVE/FREEZE GAME II

This activity continues the move/freeze idea of the Opening Activity, with more emphasis on specific movements and ending shapes. Ask the children to go to a personal space in the room. Taking ideas from any of the categories below, suggest ways that different things move and then what shape they might make when they stop their movement. Remind the children of the idea of their shape being caught in a photo.

Play a track of suggested music, such as "Sous le Soleil," softly, so that the children can hear your prompts:

1. Animals: *Let's start out by thinking of how different animals move. Examples: Hop like a frog, and then freeze like a frog catching a fly with its tongue. Move like a snake, and then coil up and freeze. Gallop like a horse, and then rear up on your back legs. Fly like a bird, and stop as if you are frozen in mid-air.*

2. Sports: *Run like a football player, and freeze like you are throwing a ball. Skate on the ice, and then balance with one leg behind. Swing a pretend baseball bat, and freeze as you watch your home run go high in the air. Pretend that you are kicking a soccer ball, and then freeze at the end of your kick. Swim as fast as you can, and freeze as you come up to take a big breath.*

3. Machines or Objects: *Move like you are inside of a washing machine, then freeze like a shirt hanging on a clothesline. Move like a bulldozer, and then freeze as you dump out a big load of dirt. Float like a bubble, and then freeze as you pop. Move like a spinning top, then freeze as you fall down.*

4. Conclude the Activity: *Did you know your body could make so many different shapes?*

How would you enhance or expand this lesson in the future?

Good-Bye Circle

With everyone standing in a circle, try this last shape dance: *Let's finish reviewing some of our favorite shapes from class. It can be one you tried, one you saw someone else make, or a new one. When I clap my hands, quickly make a shape. Now I'll clap again, and you will make your body into a different shape.* Repeat one more time, and then continue: *Now I will slowly clap three times, as you change from the first shape, to the second one, and to the third one.* (Repeat if needed until everyone can perform the sequence of the three shapes in a row.) *Now hold that last one, and bow while you are in that shape!*

Notes

What was successful about this lesson?

Which ideas could have worked better? How could they be improved?

What ideas were generated by the children during the lesson?

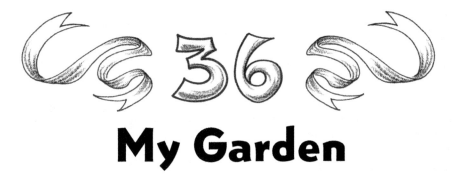

My Garden

The Carrot Seed story by Ruth Krauss provides the backdrop for a lively dance story. The children will learn what plants need in order to grow and how to tend to them as they explore the idea of growing a carrot in their own gardens.

MUSIC SUGGESTIONS:

General
- Songs or music about gardening, farms, rain, sun

Specific Selections
- "Old MacDonald Had a Farm/El Granjero" (*Uni Verse of Song: Spanish*, Maria Del Rey, Music for Little People, 1999)
- "Garden Song" (*A Child's Celebration of Song*, Various Artists, Music for Little People, 1992)
- "Mr. Sun" (*Toddler's Next Steps: Earth, Moon & Stars*, Various Artists, St. Clair Records, 2002)
- "Singin' in the Rain" (*Singin' in the Rain* (1952 Film Soundtrack), Various Artists, Rhino/Wea, 1996)

MATERIALS NEEDED:
- A small plastic watering can
- Seed packets that you can make from white paper folded and stapled into a little envelope, with a carrot drawn on the front (one for each child)
- Drum
- Optional: The book *The Carrot Seed* (Ruth Krauss, HarperCollins, 1945)

Early Learning Standards
4C, 13A, 16B

Opening Activity

Begin this class with a free dance to "Old MacDonald Had a Farm/El Granjero" (or other version) and ask the children to move like the different animals as each is named in the song. If you do not have this recorded song, you can also sing it aloud, or play another song and call out different animals that live on a farm.

Greeting Circle

Have you ever planted anything in a garden? Have you noticed how plants change as they grow?

Movement Exploration: My Garden

MOTOR SKILLS PRACTICE

Lead a warm-up of large motor skills incorporating ideas of spring and gardening:

1. Walk: *Let's take a walk through a winding garden path!*

2. March: *Let's march like we are stomping in mud puddles!*

3. Tiptoe Walk: *Tiptoe through the raindrops!*

4. Slide: *Facing your partner, make a circular shape with your arms, like a big round sun.*

5. Gallop: *Gallop through the rain! How much can we splash?*

DANCE STORY

1. Prepare for the Activity: If you have the book, read *The Carrot Seed* by Ruth Krauss. If you don't have the book, simply begin by telling the children that they will plant a garden today, using lots of imagination. Have your musical selections, the seed packets, and the watering can ready. Ask everyone to go to a personal space in the room. Prompt the children with movement as you narrate the following story:

2. Dig the Soil: *Today we are each going to plant a small garden! Find a personal space. Do you know what we have to do first? We have to dig up the soil. Get your imaginary shovel, and let's get to work!* While they are digging and planting, play "Garden Song" or another musical selection.

3. Plant the Seeds: *What do we need to do next? Plant the seeds!* Pass out the seed packets, and ask the children to plant the imaginary seeds, and then have them cover up each one with imaginary soil. Talk with the children about how the seeds need lots of sunshine in order to grow big and strong, and then ask them to place the seed packets aside.

4. Enjoy the Sunshine: Now play the song "Mr. Sun" or any other song you might have that evokes the sun, and suggest to the children that they imagine they are outside on a beautiful, sunny day, and that they dance about what it must be like to grow from a little tiny seed into a plant as the bright spring sun shines down.

5. Water the Seeds: Next ask them, *What else do plants need in order to grow? Of course, water!* Pass the empty plastic watering can around, and let each child take a turn with the can to water their seeds. After all the children have had a turn, put the watering can aside.

6. Dance in the Rain: Now the children will dance about rain. Ask them to imagine they are putting on a raincoat, rain hat, and boots, and prompt them to run outside and feel the rain on their faces. "Singin' in the Rain" is good accompaniment for this. Then suggest, *Imagine you are running and jumping in the rain, and stomping through mud puddles. Now pretend you are the rain as it falls slowly, and then very fast and hard.* Finish the dance with everyone running inside to get dry, and dry off arms, legs, head, and body with an imaginary towel.

7. Sound Improvisation: Take the next few minutes to create a little sound improvisation. Have the children return to the spot where they each "planted" their imaginary seeds. Borrowing the idea from the book *The Carrot Seed* about the little boy who is so sure his seed will come up, but everyone else doubts it, say to the children, *"We have planted the carrot seed, and it has had lots of sun and water to help it grow. But you know what? I don't think that seed you planted is going to grow!"* Encourage them to answer, *"YES IT WILL!"* Repeat this exchange several times. You can further develop this idea with nonverbal gestures, such as folded arms, head shakes, stamping feet, etc.

8. Pull Up the Carrots: Now say to the children, *Let's count to three slowly together, one . . . two . . . three! Look! A carrot plant came up! It looks like a giant carrot!*

Now let's count again, and we will pull the carrot out of the ground! Encourage the children to experiment with what it would be like to pull a very large carrot out of the ground. The same idea applies for trying to carry the big carrot. Ask, *Can you carry your big carrot around with you?* Point out to them the difference in body movements when we are carrying something very heavy versus something very light.

Good-Bye Circle:

Hold your very heavy carrot, be careful not to drop it, and take a bow to finish our dance!

Notes

What was successful about this lesson?

Which ideas could have worked better? How could they be improved?

What ideas were generated by the children during the lesson?

How would you enhance or expand this lesson in the future?

37

The Summer Night Sky

Many colorful images from the summer night sky provide creative ideas for movement. The children will explore the natural world as they imagine they are owls, fireflies, and shooting stars.

MUSIC SUGGESTIONS:

General
- Songs about night, moon, stars, the sky
- One rousing classical piece

Specific Selections
- "We're Gonna Shine," "Flyin'," and "Stardust" (*Toddler's Next Steps: Earth, Moon & Stars*, Various Artists, St. Clair Records, 2002)
- "1812 Overture" (*Tchaikovsky: 1812 Overture*, Tchaikovsky, RCA, 1991)

MATERIALS NEEDED:
- Optional: Small fiber-optic lights from a novelty store, or small flashlights (also used in Lesson 8)
- Drum

Early Learning Standards
12A, 12B, 12C

Opening Activity

For the opening activity, initiate a short discussion with the children about the night sky. Prompt them with images and ideas for movement and shapes, such as shooting stars, clouds, moon (full, half, crescent), wind, rain, owls, bats, fireflies. Play the song "We're Gonna Shine" or a similar selection about the night and ask the children to dance about the night sky.

Greeting Circle

Did you think of other things about the night sky while you were dancing? What were they? We will be dancing about all those things during today's lesson.

Movement Exploration

SEATED WARM-UP

Seated in a circle, lead the following warm-ups with night themes:

1. Body Part Isolations: *Did you know that owls sleep during the day and wake up at night? Let's be an owl, waking up in the evening. Blink your eyes open and shut. Move your head side to side, up and down, and in slow circles. Open and close your beak. Stretch your neck and shoulders! Now open and close your claws, and finally, stretch your wings. Now you are ready to go out and fly into the sky!*

2. Upper-Body Circles: Next, lead a stretch with the arms in different shapes of the moon. *Sitting with legs crossed, make a half-moon shape by lifting one arm overhead and bending the body to one side. Come back up, change arms, and bend to the other side. Then make a full-moon shape overhead, and move in an upper-body circle while holding the circle shape in the arms. Repeat, circling the upper body to the other side.*

3. Bring the Children to Standing: *Squat in a small, low shape, and then pop up to standing, pretending you are a shooting star.*

MOTOR SKILLS PRACTICE

1. Walk: *We are outside in the grass, and we want to be as quiet as possible. Shhh! How quiet can you be?*

2. Tiptoe Walk: *Let's see if we can be even quieter on our tiptoes!*

3. Run: *Next, let's pretend we are that great big owl. He will fly across the sky, and then he will swoop down when he sees something on the ground. Can you pretend to fly across the floor, swoop down, and then fly the rest of the way across the room?*

DANCE STORY: THE SUMMER NIGHT SKY

The remainder of the class will be dramatic play to a story, combining many of the nocturnal images already introduced.

1. Prepare for the Activity: Ask everyone to find a personal space. Play the song "Flyin'" or another lyrical piece for the beginning of this dance.

2. Begin the Story: *You are a little child on a beautiful summer evening. You see lots of fireflies! Dance with the fireflies!*

Now you are a sad firefly. Someone caught you and put you in a jar. You can only fly a little bit, and then you bump into the side of the jar. Try flying in all directions, but every time, you bump the side of the jar. Touch the jar, and feel the shape of it all around you. Play "Stardust" or music that is mournful or somber during this portion of the story.

3. Fiber-Optic Light Props: Pass out the fiber-optic lights or flashlights if you have brought them, change the music to the "1812 Overture" or another very lively piece, and turn out the room lights, if possible. Continue the story: *Now a child has let you out of the jar, and you are free! Fly all around the room, little fireflies!*

Suddenly, there is something even brighter and more colorful all over the sky. What do you think it is? It's fireworks! Now can you move like the fireworks, sparkling, leaping, and spreading across the clear summer night sky?

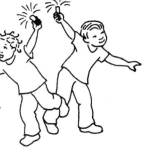

Good-Bye Circle

Let's bow with our lights on, and then turn them off all together! Or, if you do not have lights, ask the children, How would a firefly bow? Bow by flapping your wings!

Notes

What was successful about this lesson?

Which ideas could have worked better? How could they be improved?

What ideas were generated by the children during the lesson?

How would you enhance or expand this lesson in the future?

A Celebration of Movement

This class is a summation of many of the movement games and activities the children have learned and enjoyed over the course of the school year. The children will have the chance to think about all the different ways they learned to move during the year.

MUSIC SUGGESTIONS:

General
- Any music that the children have especially enjoyed throughout the year

Specific Selections
- "In the Clouds" (*Buzz Buzz*, Laurie Berkner, Two Tomatoes, 2002)
- "I've Got Imagination" (*I've Got Imagination*, Rachel Sumner, Rachel's Record, 1997)
- "When You Don't Want to Say Good-Bye" (*Dance in Your Pants*, David Jack, Ta-Dum Productions, 2002)

MATERIALS NEEDED:
- Large roll of paper, like a roll of newsprint or butcher paper
- Crayons or markers
- Tambourine
- Drum

Early Learning Standards
13A, 15A, 15B

Opening Activity: Tambourine Game

The children have been learning and dancing to rhythms throughout the year. Repeat this game from Lesson 18:

1. Review the Signals: Use your tambourine to review these signals with the children and the corresponding movements for this game. Ask the children to practice the movements as you present each signal:

March	Steady tapping on the head of the tambourine in a medium tempo
Turn	Turning the tambourine in your hands
Moving on the floor	Moving the tambourine along the floor
Gallop	Tapping faster in a gallop rhythm (LOUD-quiet, LOUD-quiet)
Run (and/or shake)	Shaking the tambourine
Hop or jump	Holding the tambourine in both hands in front of you and moving it quickly up and down
Freeze (stop cue)	One sharp, loud hit on the tambourine

2. Play the Tambourine Game: Tap a rhythm, and continue tapping it while the children perform the corresponding movement moving freely together. In between each of the movement signals, use the freeze signal to indicate a stop, before giving the next signal. Present the different signals randomly throughout the game. Finish the activity with a freeze signal.

Greeting Circle

Take some time to talk to the students about the many things they have danced about this year, and ask them to name some of their favorite activities.

Movement Exploration

1. Draw Your Favorite Movement Activities:
Unroll a long sheet of the paper and lay it along the floor so that each child has a space to work. Pass out the crayons or markers. Ask the children to take a few minutes to draw their favorites of the many things they have danced about this year. Play a musical selection such as "In the Clouds" or "I've Got Imagination" while they are drawing. When the children have finished with their drawings, display the large paper in the room.

2. Dance to Many Different Musical Selections: Play any selections of music that you have used throughout the year, and let the children dance freely about any of the ideas they have drawn on the long sheet of paper or talked about in Greeting Circle. Finish with a last dance to "When You Don't Want to Say Good-Bye" or any similar piece. The mural that the children have made can serve as a backdrop for this final dance.

Good-Bye Circle

Do you remember some of the different bows we have done this year? Do a serious bow, and then a silly bow, and then any kind of bow you wish!

Notes

What was successful about this lesson?

Which ideas could have worked better? How could they be improved?

What ideas were generated by the children during the lesson?

How would you enhance or expand this lesson in the future?

Musical Accompaniment—
Suggestions for Teachers

Four main categories of music are used throughout the book, with suggested selections below. Four CDs, one from each category, will provide plenty of musical accompaniment throughout the year.

CLASSICAL

1. *Classical Juke Box*, Vol. 1, Various Artists, Sony, 1991

2. *Classics for Kids*, Various Artists, RCA, 1993

3. *Mad about Cartoons*, Various Artists, Deutsche Grammophon, 1993

ETHNIC AND/OR UPBEAT INSTRUMENTAL

1. *The Best of World Music: World Dance Party*, Various Artists, Putumayo World Music, 1994

2. *Putumayo Presents: World Groove*, Various Artists, Putumayo World Music, 2004

3. *Bluegrass Breakdown: 14 Instrumentals*, Various Artists, Easydisc, 1997

4. *The Complete Rags of Scott Joplin*, Music Masters Jazz, 1995

CHILDREN'S SONGS

1. *Dance in Your Pants*, David Jack, Ta-Dum Productions, 2002

2. *Mother Earth*, Tom Chapin, Gadfly, 2001

3. *101 Toddler Favorites*, Various Artists, Music for Little People, 2003

4. *A Child's Celebration of Song*, Various Artists, Music for Little People, 1992

BACKGROUND MUSIC

(for the story dances and other activities that require verbal cues while the children are moving)

1. *Windham Hill 20th Anniversary Edition*, Windham Hill Records, 2001

2. *Orff-Schulwerk Vol. 1: Musica Poetica*, Carl Orff, Celestial Harmonies, 1995

3. *Celtic Awakening*, Howard Baer and Dan Gibson, 1997

Warm-Ups and Large Motor Skills

SEATED WARM-UPS

Flex and Point Feet: With legs straight ahead and together, move feet toward and away from the body.

Kitty-Cat: On hands and knees, arch and curve the back.

Merry-Go-Round: Seated with knees close to the chest, use arms to twirl the body around.

Boat: Seated with soles of feet together and knees apart, rock side to side.

Downward Facing Dog: This is a yoga position in which the body is supported equally on the hands and feet. Hands are shoulder-width apart, and feet are hip-width apart. The hips are high in the air. The knees can bend as needed.

Cobra: Lying face down, place hands flat on the floor near shoulders, with elbows close to the body. As you press the tops of the feet into the floor, breathe in and lift the chest a couple of inches off the floor. The head stays in line with the spine, and the elbows stay bent and close to the body. Slowly breathe out and lower to the floor. Repeat several times.

Lizard Crawl: Lying face down, bend to one side, and then use the hand and bent leg on that side to propel the body forward. Repeat on the other side, and continue moving forward by alternating sides.

Inchworm: On hands and knees, stretch arms and body forward and back like an inchworm.

Pill Bug: Lying on the floor on one side, curl up and stretch out several times like a pill bug. Repeat on the other side.

Upside-Down Bug: Lie on back, with arms and legs in the air.

Snow Wings: Lying face up, move arms and legs, as if to make a winged shape in the snow.

Body Part Isolations: While seated, move only one part of the body at a time, such as raising and lowering shoulders, while the rest of the body does not move.

Upper-Body Circling: Seated with legs crossed, curve the upper body to the side, continue moving until the torso is forward, and then curve to the other side, and back to the upright position, making a full circle with the torso.

Straddle Position: Sit with legs apart and back straight.

LARGE MOTOR SKILLS

Walk: Simple walks can be introduced as a way of teaching children to walk on the beat, and can be used for creative modifications and variations.

March: A modified walk, usually performed in parallel position (as opposed to the feet turning out), with knees coming up higher than in a normal walk.

Tiptoe Walk: Walking on the metatarsals, or balls, of the feet.

Lunge: A modified walk, consisting of a very large step, deeply bending the front leg while the back leg stays relatively straight.

Run: In movement classes, runs are light and quick, always with bent-knee landings.

Prance: A modified run, in which the body is held very tall. The knees are lifted and stay in front of the body, and the landing of the feet is articulated: toe, then ball, and finally the heel. The landing leg remains relatively straight—

the knee bend is very small as compared to a normal run. Prances are usually performed at a moderate speed. The image of a horse prancing is helpful in the teaching of this skill.

Gallop: A modified run, with one heavy, accented step, and a short, unaccented step. The same foot leads throughout the gallop. To beat the rhythm of a gallop: LOUD-quiet, LOUD-quiet, LOUD-quiet, GAL-lop, GAL-lop, GAL-lop.

Slide: Gallops that travel sideways. The same foot is always the lead foot in a slide, and the body faces and travels sideways. The strong beat is for the airborne part of the step, and the lighter beat is for the bent-leg landing/take-off movement. On the accented beat, the body is airborne and the following leg briefly taps or comes toward the leading leg in the air, and then lands first with a soft knee bend. The rhythm of a slide, like a gallop, is LOUD-quiet, LOUD-quiet, LOUD-quiet, SLIDE-and, SLIDE-and, SLIDE.

Jump: Two-footed jumps can be stationary (staying in one spot) or can travel in different directions. Children should always land and take off with bent knees.

Hop: One-footed hops can be stationary (staying in one spot) or can travel in different directions. Children should always land and take off with a bent knee.

Early Childhood Learning Standards: Domains, Domain Elements, and Indicators

From the Head Start Child Outcomes Framework
(Released in 2000, updated in 2003)

DOMAIN: LANGUAGE DEVELOPMENT

1. ELEMENT: Listening & Understanding

INDICATORS:

A. Demonstrates increasing ability to attend to and understand conversations, stories, songs, and poems.

B. Shows progress in understanding and following simple and multiple-step directions.

C. Understands an increasingly complex and varied vocabulary.*

D. For non-English-speaking children, progresses in listening to and understanding English.*

2. ELEMENT: Speaking & Communicating

INDICATORS:

A. Develops increasing abilities to understand and use language to communicate information, experiences, ideas, feelings, opinions, needs, questions; and for other varied purposes.*

B. Progresses in abilities to initiate and respond appropriately in conversation and discussions with peers and adults.

C. Uses an increasingly complex and varied spoken vocabulary.*

D. Progresses in clarity of pronunciation and toward speaking in sentences of increasing length and grammatical complexity.

E. For non-English-speaking children, progresses in speaking English.*

DOMAIN: LITERACY

3. ELEMENT: Phonological Awareness*

INDICATORS:

A. Shows increasing ability to discriminate and identify sounds in spoken language.

B. Shows growing awareness of beginning and ending sounds of words.

C. Progresses in recognizing matching sounds and rhymes in familiar words, games, songs, stories, and poems.

D. Shows growing ability to hear and discriminate separate syllables in words.

E. Associates sounds with written words, such as awareness that different words begin with the same sound.*

4. ELEMENT: Book Knowledge & Appreciation*

INDICATORS:

A. Shows growing interest and involvement in listening to and discussing a variety of fiction and non-fiction books and poetry.

B Shows growing interest in reading-related activities, such as asking to have a favorite book read; choosing to look at books; drawing pictures based on stories; asking to take books home; going to the library; and engaging in pretend-reading with other children.

C. Demonstrates progress in abilities to retell and dictate stories from books and experiences; to act out stories in dramatic play; and to predict what will happen next in a story.

D. Progresses in learning how to handle and care for books; knowing to view one page at a time in sequence from front to back; and understanding that a book has a title, author, and illustrator.

5. ELEMENT: Print Awareness & Concepts*

INDICATORS:

A. Shows increasing awareness of print in classroom, home, and community settings.

B. Develops growing understanding of the different functions of forms of print such as signs, letters, newspapers, lists, messages, and menus.

C. Demonstrates increasing awareness of concepts of print, such as that reading in English moves from top to bottom and from left to right, that speech can be written down, and that print conveys a message.

D. Shows progress in recognizing the association between spoken and written words by following print as it is read aloud.

E. Recognizes a word as a unit of print, or awareness that letters are grouped to form words, and that words are separated by spaces.*

6. ELEMENT: Early Writing

INDICATORS:

A. Develops understanding that writing is a way of communicating for a variety of purposes.

B. Begins to represent stories and experiences through pictures, dictation, and in play.

C. Experiments with a growing variety of writing tools and materials, such as pencils, crayons, and computers.

D. Progresses from using scribbles, shapes, or pictures to represent ideas, to using letter-like symbols, to copying or writing familiar words such as their own name.

7. ELEMENT: Alphabet Knowledge

INDICATORS:

A. Shows progress in associating the names of letters with their shapes and sounds.

B. Increases in ability to notice the beginning letters in familiar words.

C. Identifies at least 10 letters of the alphabet, especially those in their own name.*

D. Knows that letters of the alphabet are a special category of visual graphics that can be individually named.*

DOMAIN: MATHEMATICS

8. ELEMENT: Number & Operations*

INDICATORS:

A. Demonstrates increasing interest and awareness of numbers and counting as a means for solving problems and determining quantity.

B. Begins to associate number concepts, vocabulary, quantities, and written numerals in meaningful ways.

C. Develops increasing ability to count in sequence to 10 and beyond.

D. Begins to make use of one-to-one correspondence in counting objects and matching groups of objects.

E. Begins to use language to compare numbers of objects with terms such as *more, less, greater than, fewer, equal to.*

F. Develops increased abilities to combine, separate, and name "how many" concrete objects.

9. ELEMENT: Geometry & Spatial Sense

INDICATORS:

A. Begins to recognize, describe, compare, and name common shapes, their parts and attributes.

B. Progresses in ability to put together and take apart shapes.

C. Begins to be able to determine whether or not two shapes are the same size and shape.

D. Shows growth in matching, sorting, putting in a series, and regrouping objects according to one or two attributes such as color, shape, or size.

E. Builds an increasing understanding of directionality, order, and positions of objects, and words such as *up, down, over, under, top, bottom, inside, outside, in front,* and *behind.*

10. ELEMENT: Patterns & Measurement

INDICATORS:

A. Enhances abilities to recognize, duplicate, and extend simple patterns using a variety of materials.

B. Shows increasing abilities to match, sort, put in a series, and regroup objects according to one or two attributes such as shape or size.

C. Begins to make comparisons between several objects based on a single attribute.

D. Shows progress in using standard and non-standard measures for length and area of objects.

DOMAIN: SCIENCE

11. ELEMENT: Scientific Skills & Methods

INDICATORS:

A. Begins to use senses and a variety of tools and simple measuring devices to gather information, investigate materials, and observe processes and relationships.

B. Develops increased ability to observe and discuss common properties, differences, and comparisons among objects and materials.

C. Begins to participate in simple investigations to test observations, discuss and draw conclusions, and form generalizations.

D. Develops growing abilities to collect, describe, and record information through a variety of means, including discussion, drawings, maps, and charts.

E. Begins to describe and discuss predictions, explanations, and generalizations based on past experiences.

12. ELEMENT: Scientific Knowledge

INDICATORS:

A. Expands knowledge of and abilities to observe, describe, and discuss the natural world, materials, living things, and natural processes.

B. Expands knowledge of and respect for their bodies and the environment.

C. Develops growing awareness of ideas and language related to attributes of time and temperature.

D. Shows increased awareness and beginning understanding of changes in materials and cause-effect relationships.

DOMAIN: CREATIVE ARTS

13. ELEMENT: Music

INDICATORS:

A. Participates with increasing interest and enjoyment in a variety of music activities, including listening, singing, finger plays, games, and performances.

B. Experiments with a variety of musical instruments.

14. ELEMENT: Art

INDICATORS:

A. Gains ability in using different art media and materials in a variety of ways for creative expression and representation.

B. Progresses in abilities to create drawings, paintings, models, and other art creations that are more detailed, creative, or realistic.

C. Develops growing abilities to plan, work independently, and demonstrate care and persistence in a variety of art projects.

D. Begins to understand and share opinions about artistic products and experiences.

15. ELEMENT: Movement

INDICATORS:

A. Expresses through movement and dancing what is felt and heard in various musical tempos and styles.

B. Shows growth in moving in time to different patterns of beat and rhythm in music.

16. ELEMENT: Dramatic Play

INDICATORS:

A. Participates in a variety of dramatic play activities that become more extended and complex.

B. Shows growing creativity and imagination in using materials and in assuming different roles in dramatic play situations.

DOMAIN: SOCIAL & EMOTIONAL DEVELOPMENT

17. ELEMENT: Self-Concept

INDICATORS:

A. Begins to develop and express awareness of self in terms of specific abilities, characteristics, and preferences.

B. Develops growing capacity for independence in a range of activities, routines, and tasks.

C. Demonstrates growing confidence in a range of abilities and expresses pride in accomplishments.

18. ELEMENT: Self-Control

INDICATORS:

A. Shows progress in expressing feelings, needs, and opinions in difficult situations and conflicts without harming themselves, others, or property.

B. Develops growing understanding of how their actions affect others and begins to accept the consequences of their actions.

C. Demonstrates increasing capacity to follow rules and routines and use materials purposefully, safely, and respectfully.

19. ELEMENT: Cooperation

INDICATORS:

A. Increases abilities to sustain interactions with peers by helping, sharing, and discussion.

B. Shows increasing abilities to use compromise and discussion in working, playing, and resolving conflicts with peers.

C. Develops increasing abilities to give and take in interactions; to take turns in games or using materials; and to interact without being overly submissive or directive.

20. ELEMENT: Social Relationships

INDICATORS:

A. Demonstrates increasing comfort in talking with and accepting guidance and directions from a range of familiar adults.

B. Shows progress in developing friendships with peers.

C. Progresses in responding sympathetically to peers who are in need, upset, hurt, or angry; and in expressing empathy or caring for others.

21. ELEMENT: Knowledge of Families & Communities

INDICATORS:

A. Develops ability to identify personal characteristics, including gender and family composition.

B. Progresses in understanding similarities and respecting differences among people, such as genders, race, special needs, culture, language, and family structures.

C. Develops growing awareness of jobs and what is required to perform them.

D. Begins to express and understand concepts and language of geography in the contexts of the classroom, home, and community.

DOMAIN: APPROACHES TO LEARNING

22. ELEMENT: Initiative & Curiosity

INDICATORS:

A. Chooses to participate in an increasing variety of tasks and activities.

B. Develops increased ability to make independent choices.

C. Approaches tasks and activities with increased flexibility, imagination, and inventiveness.

D. Grows in eagerness to learn about and discuss a growing range of topics, ideas, and tasks.

23. ELEMENT: Engagement & Persistence

INDICATORS:

A. Grows in abilities to persist in and complete a variety of tasks, activities, projects, and experiences.

B. Demonstrates increasing ability to set goals and develop and follow through on plans.

C. Shows growing capacity to maintain concentration over time on a task, question, set of directions, or interactions, despite distractions and interruptions.

24. ELEMENT: Reasoning & Problem Solving

INDICATORS:

A. Develops increasing ability to find more than one solution to a question, task, or problem.

B. Grows in recognizing and solving problems through active exploration, including trial and error, and interactions and discussions with peers and adults.

C. Develops increasing abilities to classify, compare, and contrast objects, events, and experiences.

DOMAIN: PHYSICAL HEALTH & DEVELOPMENT

25. ELEMENT: Gross Motor Skills

INDICATORS:

A. Shows increasing levels of proficiency, control, and balance in walking, climbing, running, jumping, hopping, skipping, marching, and galloping.

B. Demonstrates increasing abilities to coordinate movements in throwing, catching, kicking, bouncing balls, and using the slide and swing.

26. ELEMENT: Fine Motor Skills

INDICATORS:

A. Develops growing strength, dexterity, and control needed to use tools such as scissors, paper punch, stapler, and hammer.

B. Grows in hand-eye coordination in building with blocks, putting together puzzles, reproducing shapes and patterns, stringing beads, and using scissors.

C. Progresses in abilities to use writing, drawing, and art tools, including pencils, markers, chalk, paint brushes, and various types of technology.

27. ELEMENT: Health Status & Practices

INDICATORS:

A. Progresses in physical growth, strength, stamina, and flexibility.

B. Participates actively in games, outdoor play, and other forms of exercise that enhance physical fitness.

C. Shows growing independence in hygiene, nutrition, and personal care when eating, dressing, washing hands, brushing teeth, and toileting.

D. Builds awareness and ability to follow basic health and safety rules such as fire safety, traffic and pedestrian safety, and responding appropriately to potentially harmful objects, substances, and activities.

* Indicates the four specific Domain Elements and nine Indicators that are legislatively mandated.

Lesson Plan Template

_____
(Lesson Title)

LESSON GOALS:

Basic Movement Skills: _____

_____

_____

Early Childhood Learning Standards: _____

_____

_____

_____

MUSIC SUGGESTIONS:

General: _____

_____

_____

Specific Selections: _____

_____

_____

MATERIALS NEEDED:

_____

_____

_____

_____

_____

LESSON DESCRIPTION:

_____

_____

_____

_____

_____

_____

_____

_____

_____

_____

_____

What was successful about this lesson? _____

_____

_____

Which ideas could have worked better? How could they be improved? _____

_____

_____

What ideas were generated by the children during the lesson?_____

_____

_____

How would you enhance or expand this lesson in the future? _____

_____

_____

Index of Lessons by Learning Domain